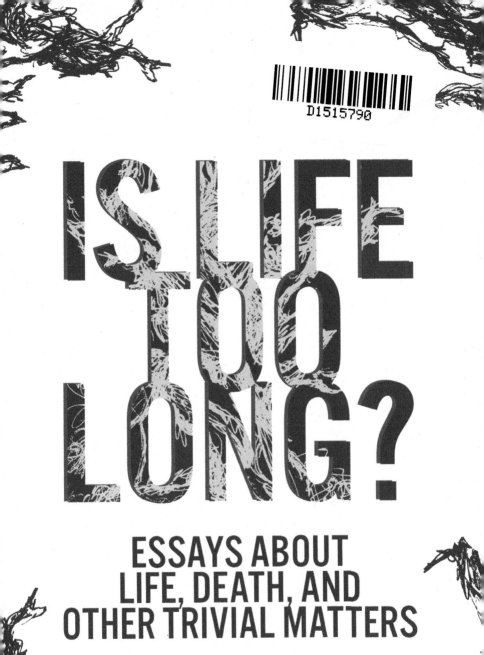

IS LIFE TOO LONG?

ESSAYS ABOUT LIFE, DEATH, AND OTHER TRIVIAL MATTERS

SHAHAR MADJAR M.D.

Is Life Too Long?
Essays About Life, Death, and Other Trivial Matters
Shahar Madjar.

Published by: Shahar Madjar, M.D.

Edited by: Dr. Shai Madjar, Florence Adar, Sharon Madjar

Text and cover design by: Guy Madjar

Illustrations by: Daniel Madjar

A CIP record for this book is available from the Library of Congress Cataloging-in-Publication Data

ISBN-13: 978-1-7328828-0-5

Contact us at: smadjar@yahoo.com

ACKNOWLEDGEMENT

I am grateful to my wife, Sharon, who was always the harshest of critics but also the most encouraging of readers; to my mother-in-law, Florence, who was instrumental in editing each of the chapters and the final version of the book; to my son, Shai, who helped editing the book and who added philosophical flavor to some of the stories, and to my sons, Guy and Danny, for giving the book its final illustrative spirit and design.

I am also grateful to a number of first readers who commented and suggested changes to the book: Dr. Ralph Horvath, Dr. Nelly G. Kupper, Dr. Moshe Wald, and Debby and Dan Wiitala.

And last, I would like to thank Stacey Willey from Globe Printing who has helped bring the book to print.

CONTENTS

INTRODUCTION

For the past several years, I have embarked on an adventure that has taken me beyond the familiar practice of medicine. I have been writing a health column. My columns, in essay format, were published every two weeks in The Mining Journal, and later in The Mining Gazette, the two leading daily newspapers of the cold, remote Upper Peninsula of Michigan.

Being a column-writer in a small town such as Marquette, the undeclared capital of the U.P., is an experience like no other. First, you get to meet your avid readers, a lot of them, everywhere you go. Second, your readers express their opinions without reservations. The image of these encounters is alive in my mind: the elderly, retired nurse who I often see at the Marquette Bakery (their Sesame Twist is heavenly) tells me that I am, at times, too philosophical; the wife of a poet who frequents Babycakes, where I take my dose of morning

Java on the weekends, offers her help with punctuation; and the greeter at the local grocery asks me to write a column about shy bladders, for he has one himself.

But, of all readers, my patients are probably the most vocal. Yes, they come to see me at my office for a first or second opinion. And, yes, they would agree to take *this* medication, drink more water, or undergo *that* operation. But, "I clipped your last week's article and sent it to my sister in Wisconsin," one patient said, and "I read your column yesterday, doctor, and I really loved it. When will your book be coming out?" asked another.

These are the people – my neighbors, my patients – who motivated me to publish a collection of my essays in a book.

But which articles should I select for the book? In what order should they appear? Should the articles have a common theme? It took me several years, and a few drafts, to make a decision. I decided to publish only the articles I love the most, in no particular order, and as a three-part series: the first book, *Is Life Too Long?* is a collection of *Essays about Life, Death, and other Trivial Matters.* I am still working on two other collections of essays: one is about love, lust, and bananas; the other is about food, my favorite subject – it will include essays on diet, health, and my recipes for an Israeli brunch extravaganza.

Several of the essays in this book describe the stories of patients, their illness, and its aftermath. These essays are all based on real events. Some of these stories are about my own patients, some are based on stories I have heard from my colleagues, and others are based on case-reports I have read in the medical literature. The names of the patients and their doctors, patients' life circumstances, the locations at which the events took place, and other identifying information have been changed to protect patient identity. In some essays, mostly those based on case-reports that were published in the medical literature, I took the liberty of creating composite characters and of adding, for dramatic effect, fictional dialogues. Although some of the facts appearing in my essays were changed, I tried to always remain loyal to the true spirit of the original stories.

This book could not have been completed without the help of a few dedicated, first readers: my dear wife, Sharon, and my mother-in-law, Florence Adar, who were always the first to opine. And my eldest son, Shai, whose strong opinions on thesis and themes have helped shape the final versions of these essays (he knows medicine, he knows philosophy, and also where every comma and period fit best).

Then my youngest son, Daniel, added his illustrations, and Guy, my middle son, gave the book its cover and its final design.

In the end, the book became a family project.

I invite you to read these essays. I hope you will enjoy reading them as much as I have enjoyed writing them.

BEETHOVEN'S EARS

People tell me that I should write what I know, so when I decided to write about Beethoven's music and his deafness, I rummaged through the drawers of my mind for a relevant memory. In an almost forgotten corner, I found a memory of myself on a wintery day in 2007, in the snowy, icy woods in the Upper Peninsula of Michigan. On that day, we were on a short, organized trip entitled "Survivorship in the Wintery Woods," or something like that. We were excited, all dressed up in multiple layers of clothing and ready to explore. Our guide, Bill (I'm sure he had no last name), had dark, scratched sunglasses and a long beard that had not met a comb for more than a decade. He took us for a long walk on a remote trail deep into the woods and asked us to walk in different directions until we could no longer see or hear each other.

I walked and walked, in the wet snow, in the cold air, until my knees hurt and the fear of losing my way back overcame my curiosity. When I stopped, I could see no one else in my group. The forest around me was white, motionless, threatening. It was also very quiet. No! Not just quiet – it was silent, completely silent! It was the closest I had ever come to being deaf.

My eerie, near-deaf experience lasted only a few seconds. It is hard to duplicate: close your eyes, cover them with an eye mask to block the light out, or enter a dark room (the kind that was used, years ago, to develop films and photographs), and you may come close, for a moment, to what a blind person experiences. But no matter how hard I press my palms against my ears, I cannot completely block out all sound.

"For the last three years," Ludwig Van Beethoven wrote to Dr. Franz Wegeler in June 1801, "my hearing has grown steadily weaker . . . I can give you some idea of this peculiar deafness when I must tell you that in the theatre I have to get very close to the orchestra to understand the performers, and that from a distance I do not hear the high notes of the instruments and the singers' voices. . . Sometimes too I hardly hear people who speak softly. The sound I can hear ... but not the words. And yet if anyone shouts I can't bear it."

Beethoven's hearing loss was progressive: in 1804, he was still able to hear conversations (and to conduct the first performance of Eroica). In 1806, he reported difficulties in hearing the woodwinds. In 1810, he reported "cotton in my ears at the pianoforte frees my hearing from the unpleasant buzzing." In 1815, Beethoven needed different hearing trumpets (the hearing aid of the time looked like a small trumpet, the narrow side of which was held close to the ear to facilitate hearing). In 1822, Beethoven reported pain on listening to instrumental music.

On May 8th, on the first performance of the Ninth Symphony, Beethoven was so deaf that he did not realize that the music had ended. One of the soloists had to physically turn him to acknowledge the public. In 1826, it is believed, Beethoven became completely deaf.

To understand Beethoven's deafness, I briefly reviewed my knowledge of the anatomy and physiology of the ear. The function of the ear, I remembered from Biology 101 class, is to convert physical vibration, or sound waves, into electrical impulses that travel through nerves. The sound waves travel through the external ear and hit the tympanic membrane, a thin membrane which is spread across the auditory canal like a taut skin over a drum. Three tiny bones shaped like a hammer, an anvil, and a stirrup conduct sound from the tympanic membrane to the inner ear. There, if you look close enough, you can find a tiny structure, about 0.2 milliliter in volume, which looks like a snail shell. It is called the "cochlea," which is ancient Greek for "spiral," or "snail shell."

It is within this tiny organ, the cochlea, that 30,000 hair cells reside, immersed in fluid. These cells specialize in translating vibration into tiny electrical signals that travel along nerve fibers into the brain.

What part of Beethoven's ear became dysfunctional? Did his ossicles become fused to the degree that they could not properly transmit vibration? Were the hair cells within his cochlea damaged? Perhaps more intriguing: What initially caused Beethoven's deafness? And how did his deafness affect his music?

When C.S. Karmody and E.S. Bachor from Tuft University School of Medicine reviewed a large number of documents written by Beethoven's contemporaries, they looked for a diagnosis that could explain not only Beethoven's deafness, but his other medical problems as well. Karmody and Bachor noticed that as a teenager, Beethoven had abdominal symptoms suggestive of inflammatory bowel disease – an autoimmune disease in which the cells of the immune system attack the patient's own body.

In inflammatory bowel disease, the main victim of the autoimmune response is the intestine, but other organs are not always spared. Unprovoked, repeated attacks of the immune system on the bile ducts inside and outside the liver can cause severe inflammation and blocking of the delicate tubes draining the liver. Eventually, failure of the liver ensues. The same autoimmune response can also cause hearing loss.

Inflammatory bowel disease, the distinguished authors conclude, was the one common thread for Beethoven's intestinal symptoms, his liver disease, his deafness, and his final demise. Was Beethoven's deafness caused by an autoimmune disease? Possibly, but unlikely, for the deafness associated with autoimmune disease progresses rapidly and is usually accompanied by vertigo. Beethoven's deafness progressed over many years, and there is no indication that he ever had vertigo.

A prescription for a mercurial compound written by one of Beethoven's physicians, Dr. Bertolini, is often used in support for another theory regarding Beethoven's deafness. The ointment, known at the time as "Volatile Salbe," was prescribed for the treatment of syphilis, which was a common disease in Beethoven's time, affecting about 15% of the world's population. Rumor has it that during a visit Beethoven paid to a prostitute, the composer contracted the thin, elongated, spiral bacteria we now call Treponema pallidum, the cause of syphilis.

Deafness did not ensue immediately, for the disease follows a predictable, protracted course, and progresses by stages: About three weeks after the alleged, unfortunate sexual encounter, Beethoven could have developed a painless, firm skin ulcer on his genitalia. Weeks later, a diffuse rash might have appeared on his trunk and on the palms of his hands and feet. The rash would be followed by a peaceful period of several years in which the composer would have no symptoms at all. The disease might then have then resurged with vengeance, affecting Beethoven's nervous system and leading, in its most severe form (called "general paresis of the insane"), to mental deterioration, personality changes and asocial behavior, depression, and at times euphoria, unexplained self-love, megalomania, and delusions of grandeur. It is in this last stage of syphilis, the theory goes, that Beethoven became deaf.

Did Beethoven contract syphilis? Was syphilis the cause of his deafness? The evidence against the syphilis theory is strong: None of Beethoven's physicians, all renowned and well versed in their contemporary medicine, ever mentioned syphilis. His deafness occurred at too young an age to be caused by advanced syphilis, and although his behavior was strange at times, and despite his greatness, he did not have delusions of grandeur.

It is not only the weakness of evidence that makes me question the syphilis theory, but also my romantic idealization of Beethoven. I refuse to believe rumors of prostitutes, Treponemas, general paresis, and insanity. I embrace a romantic Beethoven: lonely, depressed, longing, writing a sonata under the moonlight, dedicating a composition for a mysterious loved one, Fur Elise.

After the death of his mother, when he was 17, Beethoven began drinking alcohol to relieve the pain of his loss. Later, when he was thirty, he increased his wine consumption to stimulate his appetite and ease his abdominal pain. His physicians thought that he had an alcohol dependency problem, but he was not accustomed to taking medical advice seriously. Housekeeping records confirm the purchase of large quantities of wine. Ludwig preferred wine from the hills around Buda, the capital of medieval Hungary, which lies on the wooded hills west of the Danube river (the Danube river separates Buda from Pest, the two parts of the current Hungarian capital, Budapest). His personal secretary, Anton Felix Schindler, stated that Beethoven "was no judge of wine and could not tell the adulterated [wine] from the pure." It is for this reason, the theory goes, that Ludwig could not have known that his wine was tainted with lead, an additive that was illegally added at the time to improve the flavor of inexpensive wines.

Beethoven's deafness was progressive. At age 30, in a letter to a friend, Pastor Amenda, he wrote: "Know that my noblest faculty, my hearing, has greatly deteriorated." By age 47, he could no longer hear his own music.

His music did not suffer from his deafness, but it was, experts say, affected by it. In an article in the British Medical Journal, Edoardo Saccenti, Age K. Smilde, and Wim H.M. Saris, researchers from the Netherlands, charted the relations between the composer's deafness and his compositions. Analyzing Beethoven's early, middle and late string quartets, and correlating them with the three different periods in which they were written – coinciding with Beethoven's onset of deafness, worsening of hearing impairment, and the supposed total deafness – they found that a possible relation between the progression of Beethoven's deafness and the use of high notes in his music exists. The deafer he became, the less he made use of notes above high G.

At age 57, after a life afflicted by bad digestion and abdominal pain, irritability, and depression, Beethoven finally died.

Beethoven's death was not the end of Beethoven's medical story. Here is what transpired: On Beethoven's deathbed, on March 27, 1827, the great composer was visited by Dr. Ferdinand V. Hiller (a teenager at the time who admired Beethoven and later became a composer himself). After the composer's death, Ferdinand cut off a lock of hair from Beethoven's head.

The lock of hair has changed several hands: From Hiller's son to an unknown Jew. From a Danish doctor (who received it in exchange for medical care he provided for Jews trying to escape the Nazis) to members of the American Beethoven Society, who bought the lock of hair in 1994 at a Sotheby's auction for £3600. Then to Dr. Alfredo Guevera, a urologist in Nogales, Arizona. Then, of the 582 strands of hair, 422 went to Ira F. Brilliant from the Center for Beethoven Studies, and 160 were kept by Dr. Guevera. Dr. Guevera later gave a few hair strands away for the purpose of scientific investigation.

In a seemingly unrelated episode that occurred in the days following Beethoven's death, Dr. Johann Wagner, Beethoven's doctor, performed an autopsy on the body. He found a shrunken liver and ascites (both may be consistent with excessive consumption of alcohol). He closely observed Beethoven's cochlear nerves, which "lacked pith," and his acoustic nerves, which were "wrinkled." In the process, fragments from the back of the skull were separated from the body. As in Beethoven's hair story, the bone fragment must have changed several hands, for it resurfaced many years later, when a California businessman, Paul Kaufman, who inherited the bone from his great-great uncle, an Austrian doctor, submitted it for DNA analysis that confirmed that the bone contained the exact same DNA as Beethoven's hair.

In two separate, elegant studies performed by the U.S. Department of Energy's Argonne National Laboratory in 2000 and in 2005, Beethoven's bone and his hair showed markedly elevated levels of lead, consistent with chronic lead poisoning.

Was Beethoven's deafness indeed a result of lead poisoning? While some researchers are convinced by the high levels of lead found in Beethoven's hair, and in his parietal bone, others are not so sure. They bring as evidence a study of Andean children and adults with chronic lead intoxication, in which there was no hint of any harmful effect of lead on the cochlea, and no evidence of hearing loss.

As scientific evidence accumulates, the Beethoven story continues to evolve. So what was it? Was it an autoimmune disease that caused Beethoven's deafness? Syphilis? Alcohol from the hills of Buda tainted by lead? My head is spinning so hard that it is starting to ache.

I could call Bill, I think to myself, the guide from the Upper Peninsula, and ask him to take me back to the woods where complete silence fills the cold air, where I could find peace. There, I think, I could try once more to understand the meaning of silence. But could I truly understand Ludwig's deafness? I could try, I could reach, but I might never be able to truly grasp the depth of silence a deaf person experiences.

Instead, I put my headphones on and surround myself with the sounds of Beethoven's Symphony No. 9. The music, a composition written by a brilliant musician who lived in a world of silence, moves me. And I think about Beethoven, his life, and his deafness.

Can we ever truly understand the cause of Beethoven's deafness?

And I think to myself that, at times, disease and death are not the end of life's story, but merely a turning point in a medical mystery, the answer to which we will never know with certainty.

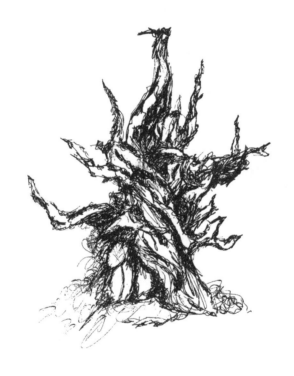

LONGEVITY

One morning, Kaylee, the receptionist at my office, declared that she is planning to work with me for the next 15 years. "Only if I live that long," I replied. "You will," she said with determination.

We often ask ourselves 'what is the meaning of life?' But as we age, many of us become interested in the simple, yet intriguing question: How long will we live?

One source attempting to address such questions is the United States government. And so, on a warm Sunday evening, in a rare moment when I had nothing else to do, I found myself visiting the Social Security website at www. SSA.gov. From a detailed table with a lot of numbers, I learned that based on my current age, I am expected to live exactly 36.12 more years.

Relieved, I wondered whether I could find different predictions if other variables were entered into the equation. What about my family history? My habits? Indeed, online longevity-calculators did require more information before they would make their final determinations. At AARP.org—the American Association of Retired Persons website—for example, I was asked about my "outlook" with questions regarding my height and weight, past medical history, and the number of days in the past month in which I was sad, depressed, or angry. They were curious about how much I move, what I eat, and how I "belong": Are you married? What is your education level? Your income? Are you satisfied at work? Do you participate in social and spiritual activities? After answering a total of 35 questions (which took me about 20 minutes), the outcome was surprisingly pleasant. According to AARP, my biological age was 8 years younger than my actual age. They gave me 13.2 years more than the government did, and said that if I lost some weight and slept more, I might live even longer, to 97.5.

I took another test at the MSN-Money website (moneycentral.msn.com), where my life expectancy was calculated to be a disappointing 73 years, and then another test at livingto100.com, where the estimate came to 90 years.

With such a diverse range of projections, I found myself swinging between hope and despair. I wondered whether my new obsession with longevity could increase the number of days in which I am sad, depressed or angry, and what effect that could have on my actual longevity.

Luckily, and quite coincidentally, a group of scientists have recently published the results of a study on longevity in the journal *Science*. Dr. Paola Sebastiani and her colleagues from Boston University School of Public Health studied DNA drawn from members of the New England Centenarian Study. The participants were not just old or elderly. They were "Well-derly," persons who lived long and well.

The researchers found genetic markers of longevity scattered along at least 70 different genes. They claim that I would soon be able to take a test that would determine whether I have the potential to live to 100 years. The test would require a complete sequence of my DNA and would cost several thousand dollars. I decided to pass.

Later, I learned that among the longest living organisms is Methuselah, the 4800-year-old bristlecone pine in California. The trunk of this ancient tree is threatening to split under the burden of life above. Another contender is the 400-year-old quahog clam (Arctica islandica) from the coast of Iceland; it does not look, at all, as happy as a clam. Finally, I looked at pictures of centenarians on Google Images and I saw wrinkled faces and hard-earned wisdom. Suddenly I started to doubt the benefits of extreme longevity.

After a good night's sleep and a healthy breakfast, I returned to my satisfying workplace. I told Kaylee that I checked several sources and that I am expecting to live at least several more decades. I explained that based on my projected longevity, I will probably never be able to retire, and therefore her job is secure for at least 15 years, just as she wanted. "I told you so last week," she said as she brought a patient into Exam Room 1. "Now we have to work!"

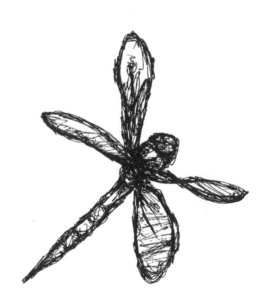

DRAGONFLY

Once every two years I travel to my home country, Israel. I usually stay in Tel Aviv, where it is almost always summer, and the days are long and hot. I enjoy sitting in a cafe along the beach, and I watch the waves of the Mediterranean Sea as they break on the shore. The air carries a thin mist of steam and salt. I feel the hot sand between my toes. I order a strong, sweet coffee which the locals call *Botz* (mud) and a feast the locals call an Israeli Breakfast. I people-watch, and I listen: to the sounds of the waves breaking in the distance, to the lifeguard calling the swimmers to stay out of the deep water and away from turbulent currents, to the sound of wooden paddles hitting a small rubber ball in an endless game called *Matkot*. The pairs of players, I notice, pass the ball with energy and speed, trying to disprove the rules of gravity. When they fail, when the ball falls into the sand, they sound surprised and blame each other; then, they laugh a little and keep playing.

I also listen to conversations at the tables around me. I do not eavesdrop, but I happen to hear – bits and pieces, not whole conversations.

On my last visit to Israel, I was sitting in the cafe, and I was listening. Everyone was talking about love, or food, or politics. People were saying: "It is so hot today," or "he is so handsome," or "this breakfast is delicious," or "Bibi (the prime minister, Benjamin Netanyahu) is doing a good job."

I listened to all of these statements, and I immediately thought: *Compared to what?*

I asked 'compared to what?' without criticism for my fellow human beings who utter these statements, for I, too, have made such statements without considering the possible comparisons. There were times, for example, that I have said, or rather quoted others who have said "life is too short to be unhappy." Things like that.

'No longer!' I resolved. From now on, every statement would be accompanied with a comparison. I decided to start with a simple question: Is life too short?

And I immediately responded: Too short? Too long? Compared to what?

In the *Compton's Pictured Encyclopedia,* published in 1939, I found a picture that is worth more than a thousand words. It is called: *How Long Do Animals Live?* The picture drawn by Gerd Arntz shows more than three dozen animals as they stand along a serpentine line. They are arranged in order of their longevity. At the beginning of the line is a small drawing of an insect, a short-lived, feeble creature drawn in yellow; farther along the line is a rat and a mouse. The insect, the rat, and the mouse all live less than five years. Then, a hare, a toad, and a fox. A lion and a woodpecker take a more fortunate position, living between 10 and 15 years. And as my eyes traveled downwards along the diagram, I saw a dog, an elk, then a crocodile (with sharp teeth and no tears, the crocodile almost reaches the 25-year mark). Then, a hippopotamus leads the way, just in front of a crane, and lives very close to 40 years. An elephant of about 60 years is then depicted in red, his tusks pointing forward. Then a whale (70). And far down the wandering line, one can see the giant tortoise, which lives, slowly yet steadily, to 150 years.

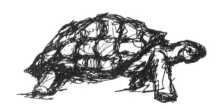

Gerd Arntz's picture is vivid and beautiful. The animals along the line are drawn as simple silhouettes in yellow, red, black, and blue (for invertebrates, mammals, birds, and other vertebrae, respectively). Looking at Gerd Arntz's picture, the kid that lives in me jumps up and down with curiosity and happiness, as if I have just discovered a new continent.

Then comes the critical me: I somberly think, for example, that grouping all insects into a tiny, yellow *insect* picture is an atrocity against insects, entomologists, and anyone interested in longevity. After all, a termite queen can live to 50 years, a spider lives for 2 years, a mosquito lives just a little more than a month, and the common fly lives for 15-25 days. Even among the insects we call moths, variation rules.

Variation? I ask myself, what variation? I just *know* that the life of a moth is short, for I am not afraid of Virginia Woolf. In her essay, The Death of a Moth, I found sentences like: "One was, indeed, conscious of the queer feeling of pity for him [the moth]. The possibilities of pleasure seemed that morning so enormous and so various that to have only a moth's part in life... appeared a hard fate, and his jest in enjoying his meager opportunities to the full, pathetic."

As she observed the moth dying, Virginia Woolf noticed that "The body relaxed, and instantly grew still. The struggle was over. The insignificant little creature knew death... O yes, he seemed to say, death is stronger than I am." For Virginia Woolf, the moth's struggle for its life is the struggle of all living creatures, of us all, a reflection on her own life's struggles and of her upcoming death. On March 28, 1941, Woolf filled her overcoat pockets with stones and walked into the River Ouse near her home in Lewes, Sussex, England. She drowned. *The Death of a Moth and Other Essays* was published in 1942.

Would Virginia Woolf have written *The Death of a Moth* if she knew that the life of a moth is not as short as she had believed? The life span of the brown house moth, for example, is quite variable, and some brown house moths live, if one takes into account the incubation period and the larval stage, for up to 13 months!

As I examine Gerd Arntz's picture and admire its simplicity and beauty, I notice not only generalization and imprecision, but omission. I carefully look again, and nowhere along the serpentine line is a depiction of the species to which I belong. Yes! Homo sapiens, (Latin for "wise man," although not all members equally merit the title) is missing from Arntz's *How Long Do Animals Live?*

The concept of life expectancy is difficult to grasp, partly because your life expectancy is a moving target—it changes as you grow older.

In the USA, for example, life expectancy at birth is 78.94

years. This means that if you were to be born today, you would be expected to live until you are 78.94. Women live longer while men have a shorter life expectancy (81.05 vs. 76.28 years, according to the Social Security Period Life Table).

As you get older, your life expectancy decreases—you simply have fewer years to live. For a woman in the USA, for example, life expectancy at birth is 81.05, at age 18 it is 63.68 years, and at 65, life expectancy is 20.32 years.

Here is some good news, though: while your life expectancy decreases with every passing year, your expected age at death increases! So, in the example above, a 65-year-old woman is expected to live until she is 85.32, which is higher than her life expectancy at birth.

This sounds somewhat counter-intuitive, but consider the 65-year-old woman in the example above: she did not die of sudden infant death, she did not drown in her parents' pool at age 4, she didn't commit suicide because of unrequited love at age 18, she did not succumb to breast cancer at 58, nor to a deadly heart attack or a lethal stroke at 64. She survived all of these and many other events that could have resulted in her earlier demise. She entered a group of older people who avoided earlier death, and are expected, at least statistically, to live longer.

Is life too short? 78.94 years—the life expectancy at birth in the USA—sounds like a good number of years, except, of course, if you just celebrated your 77th birthday.

But how does life expectancy compare in different parts of the world? The World Factbook of the Central Intelligence Agency (CIA) reports that Monaco leads the way with a life expectancy of 89.5 years (my mother told me I should marry the princess of Monaco; I never listen). Singapore follows (85 years). Italy is at the 14th location (82.2). Israel is ranked 11th (82.4), and Canada and France are at the 19th and 20th places (81.9, 81.8). Finland is ranked 31st (80.9 years).

The United States, according to the CIA, is ranked at the 42nd spot (79.8, 2016 estimate), which may sound disappointing, unless you consider the other 182 countries on the list: Denmark (life expectancy is 79.4), Hungary (75), Yemen (65), and further down the list is Afghanistan (51.3), and last, at the 224th spot, is Chad, where a newborn is expected to live a mere 50.2 years.

When talking about life expectancy, one should consider not only geography, but history. We live longer than ever: In classical Greece, life expectancy was 28 years. In the late medieval England (5th to 15th centuries), it was 30 years, because the Great Famine and Black Death killed about half of England's population. In 1900, the world average life expectancy was 31. And not so long ago, in 1950, it was 48. Compared to prior generations, we live in a time of long life.

Back in the USA, at work, during an unexpected break between patients, I found myself taking a short walk in nature. There, behind the hospital, lies a small pond surrounded by trees. As I was in the habit of making comparisons, I noticed that I was in a place unlike any other, in God's country. I was completely alone, or so it seemed. And the silence was disturbed only by the chirping of birds and the remote sounds of traffic on US-2.

Then, out of somewhere, came a dragonfly. It flew with vigor and purpose, making circles around me and a statement: this pond is mine! The life of a dragonfly, I thought, is short—shorter than mine by a lot, for it was, after all, just an insect—but I felt no pity, for its part in life, short or long, seemed as complete as that of any other member of Nature's creatures, and filled with a passion for living.

LIGHT AT THE END OF THE TUNNEL

And at the end of life, yet another transition awaits: from life to death, from being to being no more. What happens at the twilight zone, just before life ends, is an interesting question. And attempts to better understand this 'near-death experience' have always drawn the attention of curious minds.

Before I dwell on the recent attempts made by the scientists to address the phenomenon of near-death experience, I wanted to tell you about a Russian writer by the name of Lev Tolstoy. Yes, he wrote 'Anna Karenina', and 'War and Peace', but much more relevant to our discussion is his novella 'The Death of Ivan Ilyich'. Tolstoy's characters suffer from palpable pain, heart-wrenching grief, and tremendous misery. In short, they experience a very Russian existence. And such is the story of Ivan Ilyich, who at the age of 45 developed an incurable and painful disease. His pain was excruciating, his suffering unimaginable. Desperate, he sought medical advice, but "it was all as he expected, it was all as it was always done. The waiting and the assumed doctorly importance..." Diagnoses such as a floating kidney and appendicitis were triumphantly made. Later, "Ivan Ilyich drew the conclusion that things were bad," and in the end, there was no relief, no cure. He realized that he was not merely ill, he was dying.

'The Death of Ivan Ilyich' ends, how surprising, with Ivan Ilyich's death. The book is short, but Ivan's painful death is studied in detail as if it was a scientific journey into the soul of a dying man. And what exactly was the near-death experience Ivan Ilyich had? Tolstoy writes: Ivan Ilyich "sought his own habitual fear of death and could not find it. Where was it? What death? There was no more fear because there was no more death. Instead of death *there was light*... He drew in air, stopped at mid-breath, stretched out, and died."

The attempts to solve the mystery of the last moments of life did not end with Tolstoy, nor did it end with the demise of his fictional character, Ivan Ilyich. More than 100 years after the publication of 'The Death of Ivan Ilyich', a group of Dutch scientists set to investigate the experiences of 344 patients that were successfully resuscitated after their hearts had stopped beating. Doctors call it cardiac arrest. Out of this group, 62 patients (18%) reported 'near-death experience' with at least some recollection of the time of their death. Most patients reported that they remember having positive emotions, half of the patients reported being aware of themselves being dead, and several patients reported out of body experience, moving through a tunnel, observation of colors or of celestial landscape, and meeting with deceased persons. But more interestingly, fourteen patients (23%) had experiences similar to the one described by Tolstoy, whereby they had "communication with light."

More recently, a group of scientists from the University of Michigan went even further in their quest to understand near-death-experiences. In their experiment, they studied adult rats. They served the rats food and water and let them acclimate to their new home at the laboratory. Then they put the rats under anesthesia and implanted electrodes in their hearts, and into the cortex of their brains. They fixed the electrodes to the rats' skulls using dental glue. Then they injected potassium chloride solution into the rats' hearts, inducing their death. What followed was a surprise: at their last moments of life, the rats' brains was not quieting down or shutting off. On the contrary, their brain activity was surging, producing oscillations that were "global and highly coherent."

The scientists from Michigan then took a far-reaching leap to humans and their near-death experience: "We now provide," they wrote "a scientific framework to begin to explain the highly lucid and realer-than-real mental experiences reported by near-death survivors." And the poetic and compassionate description of near-death experience by Tolstoy became a simple current of minute electrical impulses.

If life is a series of consequential transitions, then at the end of life, yet another transition awaits. When my time comes, I would rather my last vision of life be described by a writer, not by a scientist.

IS LIFE TOO LONG?

Is life *really* too short? Some prominent doctors claim that life is too long.

Dr. Ezekiel J. Emanuel, a professor at the University of Pennsylvania School of Medicine and Chair of the Department of Ethics and Health Policy, wants to die at 75. In an article published in *The Atlantic,* he wrote: "Death is a loss ... but living too long is also a loss." By age 75, Ezekiel claims, he would have lived a full life: he would have loved and been loved, he would have pursued his life's projects, and he would have done so without too many mental and physical limitations.

The productive, creative years, Ezekiel claims, end at an age much younger than 75. There are exceptions, of course, but the average age at which Nobel Prize winning physicists make their discoveries is 48; classical composers peak at about 40. He speculates that the age-creativity connection is biological in nature: In older persons, new sets of neural connections just don't form as easily as they did in a younger age. I ask myself: is a life of bursting creativity, of intense productivity, the only life worth living?

As we age, Ezekiel writes, "We accommodate our physical and mental limitation. Our expectations shrink ... we are aspiring to and doing less and less." He writes that as he or she grows old, the American immortal – a term he uses to describe a person engaged in a valiant effort to cheat death and prolong life as long as possible – is happy to cultivate avocational interests: taking up bird watching, poetry and the like... I ask myself: what is wrong with poetry, the like, or an occasional session of bird-watching?

In a final attempt to sell a shorter life, Dr. Ezekiel turns to our conscious and to our deep desire to leave an impeccable, long-lived legacy: by living too long, the elderly become "a very real and oppressive" financial and caregiving burden. And while we want to be remembered by our children and grandchildren as active, engaged, funny, warm, and loving, by living too long, Ezekiel writes, we risk being remembered as sluggish, forgetful, stooped.

As I thought about the elderly people I knew, I realized that the sluggish, forgetful, stooped image of them aging would never overshadow my memories of them as their engaged, warm, loving younger selves. I did not feel burdened by the need to care for older people, but privileged to share time with them. Observing men and women clinging to life, I realized how intense, how deeply natural is the drive to live. By knowing them, I gained a new appreciation for the finality of life, for its value – life is too short, I immediately concluded. Live life to its fullest.

Dr. Ezekiel was not the first to prescribe the not-too-long life. Almost a century before the publication of 'Why I Hope to Die at 75', another renowned physician, Sir William Osler, presented the same ideas, with a twist. Osler was a Canadian physician, a respected medical educator, an author, and a bibliophile, a founding father of the Johns Hopkins Hospital, and later the Chair of Medicine at Oxford University, England. He was well known in the medical community and to the general public. Diseases, signs and symptoms were named after him. And so, when he delivered his famous—or infamous—speech called 'The Fixed Period', people listened.

"Take the sum of human achievement in action, in science, in art, in literature – subtract the work of men above 40, and while we should miss great treasures, even priceless treasures, we would practically be where we are today," Osler said as he expanded on the theme of the energy of youth and the uselessness of old age. In that same speech, he recommended that men retire at age 60. Then, apparently jokingly, he added: "Whether Anthony Trollope's suggestion of ... chloroform [for the elderly] should be carried out or not I have become a little dubious, as my own time is getting so short.".

Newspapers, magazines, doctors, and the general public reacted to Osler's words swiftly. His claims regarding the worthlessness of old men were intensely disputed. The Louisville Monthly Journal of Medicine and Surgery came out with the headline 'Osler's nonsense'. Others said he was 'heartless'. And a senator from Nevada called him 'a crank'.

Is life really too long? Medicine can extend and improve life well beyond 40, 60, even 75 – cataract surgery and hearing aids will make you see and hear the world, artificial hips and knees will get you going, prostate surgery will keep you flowing, Viagra will keep you proud, and coronary artery stents and open-heart surgery will keep the blood streaming in your arteries. But is all of this effort worthwhile?

But what if life is a story in search of an ending? What if life needs to last longer – beyond 75, 80, 85 – just for the narrative of life to reach a conclusion? I rummaged in my memory for such stories and found several.

Consider Dr. Henry Heimlich's story: in 1974, at age 54, the thoracic surgeon described a maneuver that has since been adapted worldwide as the standard response to a choking victim. In an article published in Emergency Medicine, he wrote: "Each year in the United States, 3,900 healthy people strangle on food stuck in their tracheas ... The incident generally occurs at a dinner table. The victim suddenly chokes, turns blue or black, and is dead in minutes." Dr. Heimlich then described a simple solution: stand behind the victim, put both arms around him just above the belt line, grasp your right wrist with your left hand and rapidly and strongly press into the victim's abdomen. This, Heimlich suggested, would force the diaphragm upward, compress the lungs and expel the obstructing bolus.

In May 2016, at age 96, Heimlich used his own maneuver and saved Patty Gill Riss, 87, who sat next to him in the dining room at a senior living community in Cincinnati, Ohio. She started to choke. He stood up, spun the woman around, and performed his namesake maneuver. Patty coughed out a piece of hamburger. In a picture taken after the event, Heimlich and Riss are seen smiling from ear to ear. "Thank this wonderful man for saving my life," she said. They seem happy and excited, ready to write yet another chapter in the narrative of their lives.

Then, consider another story that took place an ocean away: The sisters Sarah and Hannah Tesler were born on the same day, three years apart. Always together, never separated from each other, they survived the Auschwitz concentration camp. The sisters shared two dreams: the first, to immigrate to Israel, and to build their home and bring up their families there. Sarah and Hannah fulfilled their first dream in Kibbutz Yavne, in the lush coastal plains of Israel. Their second dream, to donate a Torah scroll to the local synagogue commemorating their family members who were killed in the holocaust, had to wait longer. They introduced their gift, hand-written Torah scrolls, in 2015, on their 87th and 90th birthdays.

The two stories are not only touching, they also seem to confirm the theory that life is a story in search of an ending, that life needs to last longer – beyond 75, 80, 85 – just for the narrative of life to reach a conclusion, or better yet, a happy ending.

Just as I was preparing to complete my article with this cheerful notion, reality hit me hard, for I suddenly recalled other stories that disprove this theory. One story in particular came to my mind:

Mr. H., a patient of mine from Stony Brook, NY, was diagnosed with bladder cancer. He was in his eighties, hard of hearing, but still in reasonably good shape. His cancer, though, was severe and complicated. Mr. H. wanted to live longer and was willing to submit himself to chemotherapy. On a winter day, as he was driving to his chemotherapy session ("it was a snowy day," he told me later, "and the snow hit the windshield so hard that I could barely see a thing"), Mr. H. hit a young woman with his car. She died hours later. I saw Mr. H. several days after the accident took place. He stood in front of me, stricken by guilt, tears in his eyes. "I should have died earlier," he told me.

Is life too short? Too long? As I was looking for answers, I stumbled upon *Gratitude*, a book of four short essays written by Oliver Sacks. At age 82, after he had learned that his rare form of melanoma of the eye had metastasized to his liver, Sacks wrote: "My predominant feeling is one of gratitude. I have loved and been loved, I have been given much and have given something in return; I have read and traveled and thought and written... Above all, I have been a sentient being, a thinking animal, on this beautiful planet, and that in itself has been an enormous privilege and adventure."

Life is too short for some, too long for others. For the most fortunate, life is a story just long enough to find a good ending, to gain perspective, and to patiently learn the art of gratitude.

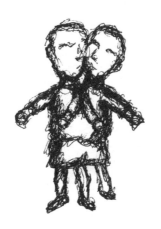

THE TWINS' DILEMMA

When the twins were born, there was little reason to celebrate. Their mother, Faith, noticed that her friends were no longer coming to visit. She noticed that people around her were whispering to one another. When she asked them what they were saying, they sometimes refused to repeat themselves, and on other occasions they came up with something not worth whispering about. She knew that they were talking about the twins and about her, that they were avoiding her and the twins as if the condition were contagious. At night, Faith cried. And when she went to the hospital for consultation, one doctor explained that such things just happened. Faith thought she heard him saying, "It is an accident of nature."

The twins were conjoined.

At 22 months, Faith brought the twins to a hospital where doctors specializing in separating conjoined twins examined them.

The twins had two heads that were facing each other. They had two chests. But they were attached to each other from the xyphoid bone to the pelvis. They had only one belly button, one anus, and one vagina. They had four arms, but only three legs. One of the legs had a duplicated foot with seven toes: one large toe in the middle, and three smaller toes on each side.

Faith read online that conjoined twins are extremely rare. That the chance is 1 in 100,000 births. "Why does it have to be me?" she thought. She read that most conjoined twins are either stillborn or die within the first day of their life. When her spirit was broken, she wondered whether it would have been better if her twins had died too. At other moments, though, she was prepared to fight for the twins' lives against all odds.

She read that conjoined twins are formed when a fertilized egg fails to completely split in the middle. If her twins had completed the split, they would have been separate, but hers were of the incomplete-split type, and so were joined together.

Faith read that conjoined twins are always identical. Her girls looked similar, but one of the girls was larger, and always seemed more lively—she laughed louder and was more eager to play.

When the doctors looked at the CAT scan images of

the twins, they found that the twins shared a single, long liver. Each twin had only one functioning kidney and a single ureter (the tube that drains the urine from the kidneys to the bladder). The ureters were draining into one common bladder. A part of the intestine was partially fused and another part was common to both twins.

The larger twin had an almost normal heart anatomy.

The smaller twin had severe heart disease. Her heart could not support her own needs. Her life was dependent on her sibling's circulation.

The lips of the smaller twin were blue, and her oxygen levels were low. Several days after she arrived in the hospital, the smaller twin developed fever and appeared tired. She was less active than usual, she cried faintly, and her nails turned blue. She coughed all the time. She initially responded to antibiotics, but soon thereafter her condition deteriorated again.

Without surgical intervention, it was likely that the smaller twin would die and that the death of the smaller twin would lead to the death of the healthier one.

Should the doctors intervene by performing surgery to separate the twins?

The answer seems simple when the question is formulated in mathematical terms: the twins are two persons. Doing nothing will most likely result in the death of both girls. Surgically separating the twins will most likely result in the death of one twin and the survival of the other. And since one life is better than none, surgery should be performed.

But the question, you see, may not be one of numbers. Would it be ethical, after all, to take an action that we know would most likely end the life of one of these children? Can the saving of one life justify the ending of the other? And who should be making these kinds of decisions?

What should the surgeons do? What did the surgeons decide to do? Were the lives of the girls saved?

No matter how hard she tried, Dr. Margaret Wise could not suppress the image of the fat man standing on the bridge.

She had learned about the fat man as a medical student, during Bioethics 101, a class she elected to take in the summer semester of 1991.

Dr. Wise remembered the lesson vividly. The bioethics professor, a man with a long beard and round, black glasses stood in front of a group of students and described the problem – he called it the Trolley Problem – as such:

Suppose you are standing along the side of a railway track. A trolley is coming down the track. Ahead, there are five people tied up to the track. They are unable to free themselves, and there is no one that can help them escape. Without any intervention, the trolley would run over the five people, and they would die. Now, *you* are standing a few steps from the track next to a lever. If you pull the lever, the trolley will be diverted onto a different track where there is only one person tied up.

"What would *you* do?" The professor asked the students.

Margaret initially thought that the Trolley Problem was not difficult: If she did nothing, the five people tied to the main track would die. If she pulled the lever, diverting the trolley onto the side track, only one person would die. Pulling the lever and saving the lives of five people, she thought, would be the most appropriate action.

"But what if," the professor asked – the way philosophers do when they want to prove that the initial response to a problem is not necessarily the most appropriate ethical solution – "what if the person tied to the different track is of particular value to society, say a beloved leader, a doctor who can save the lives of many, or an artist whose works inspire millions of people ... or, what if the person tied to the different track is your beloved father, your sister, your son? Would you still divert the trolley?"

The classroom fell silent. And Margaret was not so sure anymore.

"Let's complicate the problem even more," the professor said as he introduced the fat man dilemma. "Imagine a similar situation: the trolley is moving along the track toward five people tied to the track. But there is no other track this time, and no lever! Instead, you are standing on a bridge over the track. Next to you stands a very fat man. You can push the fat man off the bridge and onto the track. The fat man would definitely die, but his heavy body would ultimately stop the trolley and save the five people tied to the track. Would you push the fat man onto his death, in order to save the lives of five people?

Margaret knew that although the arithmetic of the two situations was similar – after all, in both situations it was a choice between five lives and one life – she could not push the fat man to his death.

"Not so simple anymore, huh?" The professor laughed briefly.

"Now consider an even more difficult dilemma," the professor continued. "Suppose you are already a doctor, and suppose there are five patients waiting for a transplant. One of them needs a heart transplant, two need a kidney, another needs a liver, yet another needs a lung transplant. Without a transplant, they would all die. During the course of your day, you examine a young man who you see for a routine checkup. You find out that he is not only in perfect health, but he would be a perfect donor for all five patients. Suppose the man is just a drifter that passes through town. He has no family and no friends, and should he disappear, nobody would inquire about him. Would you support killing the drifter to save the lives of the five people in need of transplantation?"

Years later, on the night before an ethics committee meeting, Dr. Wise could not fall asleep. The image of the fat man on the bridge kept appearing in her mind. And so did the image of the bioethics professor with his trolleys and the unaccounted-for drifter whose theoretical murder could really save lives. She knew that tomorrow, at the ethics committee, she would be faced with a real case: the case of conjoined twin girls attached to each other from the xyphoid bone to the pelvis. One is well; the other is sick, but still alive. Doing nothing will most likely result in the death of both girls. Surgically separating the twins would most likely result in the death of one twin and the survival of the other. Would sacrificing one twin in order to save the other be justified?

Dr. Wise tried to tune out the image of the fat man. She sank into her bed, and her eyes closed. Tomorrow is a big day, she thought, just before she fell asleep – time for decision.

The hospital ethics committee convenes monthly, on Mondays, at 7:00 AM sharp. The committee meets on the 12th floor of the hospital. There are seven members: 3 doctors, a lawyer, a priest, a bioethicist, and a representative of the community. Dr. Wise is the chairperson.

Dr. Wise knew the committee members' love for endless philosophical debates. She also knew that the case that she would present on that particular Monday – the twins' dilemma – required a timely decision.

Dr. Wise presented the case of the conjoined twin girls: "The twins were admitted to the hospital a week ago. They are conjoined. One of the twins is well; the other is sick, but still alive. Doing nothing would most likely result in the death of both girls. Surgically separating the twins would most likely result in the death of one twin and the survival of the other. Can we proceed with a surgery to separate the twins?" She asked.

The committee members looked at the pictures of the twins and the images that were obtained at the radiology department. The twins had two heads that were facing each other. They had two chests. But they were attached to each other from the xyphoid bone to the pelvis. They had four arms, but only three legs.

"A real problem," one of the members said. "Awful," another member agreed.

"We believe it is surgically possible to separate the twins," a doctor from the Department of Pediatric Surgery said.

"The real question is whether sacrificing one twin in order to save the other could be justified," the bioethicist said.

"But if doing nothing will most likely result in the death

of both girls, and surgically separating the twins will most likely result in the death of only one, isn't it better to separate them?" Sara, the community representative asked.

"Imagine a similar situation," the priest said, "in which the twins are not conjoined, but separate. So, we would have two twin sisters. One of the sisters is smaller, and very sick, but her heart is functioning well. The other sister is healthy except she has severe heart disease. Would you support sacrificing the smaller, very sick twin with the good heart to save the life of the other twin. Would that be justified?"

Sara was not so sure anymore. There was silence first, then an animated debate that led nowhere. The time was 7:45. The twins, their mother, and the surgeons were waiting for a decision.

Dr. Wise looked at Sara, at the priest, and at the other members of the committee. "So what is the right thing to do? What is the moral thing to do? Perhaps," she said, "it is time to apply the four principles of bioethics." The bioethicist nodded. The committee members agreed. They reviewed the case in light of these principles:

Beneficence, or the intent to do good for the patient: in the conjoined twins' case, surgery would most likely result in a longer life to the healthier twin.

Non-maleficence, or the intent to not harm the patient: surgery may result in the early death of the sicker twin and could potentially harm the healthy twin.

Respect for Autonomy, or the intent to respect the patient's decision: the twins cannot make a decision regarding their medical treatment. Their mother could, though, and her wish should be considered and honored.

Justice, or the intent to provide fair distribution of medical resources: because of the great expense of surgery and its uncertain results, it is not clear whether this treatment is justified.

And there were perhaps other ethical considerations: the wish of the twins themselves (if they could tell us their wish); the true intent of the medical intervention; the morality of acting vs. letting nature take its course.

The committee discussed these principles and considerations. The mother expressed her wish to proceed with the surgical separation of the twins. The committee decided that the mother's wish and the benefit to the healthier twin outweighed the cost of harm done to the sicker child, who would have died anyway.

The surgery was technically challenging. It took several surgeons from different specialties and 14 hours to separate the twins. As expected, the smaller twin died during surgery.

The larger twin survived the operation. After several weeks of recuperation, she was able to crawl and stand with assistance. Her doctor believed that she would do well.

On her way home, on the airplane, Faith, the mother of

the twins, held her baby close to her chest. The twin was sleeping, her eyes closed. "So precious," Faith whispered as she passed her hand over the twin's hair, "my baby, you are so precious."

Dr. Wise and the ethics committee are scheduled to meet again on the upcoming Monday, at 7:00 AM sharp. On the agenda, there is another case to discuss.

DORA MARR AND CAT

A Chinese doctor is growing an ear on a patient's arm, and all I can think about is Dora Maar and her cat.

The Chinese physician is Dr. Guo Shuzhong, a plastic surgeon from a hospital in Xi'an Jiaotong University. His patient, Mr. Ji, lost his right ear in a car accident. "I lost one ear. I have always felt that I am not complete," Mr. Ji told the China News. Dr. Guo Shuzhong decided to create a new ear for Mr. Ji. He first inserted a skin expander, an inflatable balloon device, into the arm of the patient. Then he injected water into the expander to increase its volume and stretch the overlying skin. He then took three pieces of cartilage from the patient's chest, carved them into the shape of an ear, and inserted them into the newly created space.

Mr. Ji and Dr. Guo Shuzhong are waiting for the ear to grow. In a few months, the ear will be harvested from Mr. Ji's arm and transplanted to his head.

The image of an ear growing in Mr. Ji's arm reminds me of Dora Maar. Dora Maar was born Henriette Theodora Markovitch in 1907, in Paris. She was a photographer, painter, poet, and the lover and muse of Pablo Picasso. He was 55, she was 29, love bloomed, then things got complicated: he painted her as a weeping woman (several times), described her as an Afghan cat, and painted her again and again, in convoluted, tortured forms.

In a 1941 painting, Dora Marr au Chat (Dora Maar with Cat), Dora is sitting on a chair like a queen on her throne. She is wearing a hat that sits on her head like a crown. Behind Dora's right shoulder, on the top rail of her chair, a black cat is standing – I can't see the cat's eyes, but I feel that it is looking at me. Dora wears red and green, blue and purple. Dora's arms are resting on the armrests, her long fingers curled around the arms of the chair; her nails are sharp, black and violent.

But more concerning for the innocent art-lover is Dora Maar's face. As in Mr. Ji's story, where an ear somehow finds its way to an arm, things are just not where they're supposed to be. Dora's left eye is hanging just above the mouth in the middle of her face, and the left ear is touching the left eye. The nose has shifted all the way to the right side of Dora's face, and it looks like it has a smaller face of its own – I can see at least one eye, an eyebrow, and a nostril. Dora's mouth is the only part that stayed in place – relatively speaking, that is.

Doctors and artists seem to be taking the liberty of moving things around. I saw it first-hand when I learned, more than a decade ago, during a fellowship at the University of Miami, that injuries to the urinary system can be treated by harvesting tissue from the inner-cheek lining (buccal mucosa) and transferring it to the urethra (the tube through which we urinate). My mentor at the time was Dr. Angelo Gousse. We were operating on a man who was kicked in the groin during a fight in a Miami bar several years prior. During the months that followed, the man developed scar tissue at the site of injury, along his urethra, causing severe blockage and constricted flow of urine. In surgery, we kept the patient's mouth open using a special retractor and harvested a small strip of buccal mucosa. We then made an incision along the scarred area in the urethra. We stitched the buccal mucosa into the edges of our longitudinal incision, the way seamstresses expand the waistband of pants by opening at the seams and adding fabric to the waistline. The patient fared well. Several weeks after his surgery, when he returned to our clinic, the wound in his inner cheek seemed healed. And he, a farmer by profession, proudly announced: "I pee like a horse!"

I wish Mr. Ji a successful relocation of his ear to his head, and I hope that he will feel complete again. As for Dora Marr, Picasso ended their relationship, replacing her with Francoise Gilot, another lover and muse. Dora suffered frequent bouts of depression and lived reclusively in the shadow of the image Picasso had created for her. She died in 1997 in her Left Bank apartment in Paris. She was 89.

Dora Marr au Chat was sold at a Sotheby's auction in London to an anonymous buyer for $95,216,000. It is on the list of the most expensive artworks ever sold.

JUST A CUT

When it comes to ill-wishes, people can get really creative. For example, one Yiddish insult translates to, "I hope you swallow an umbrella, and that it opens up in your stomach." And another says, "May all of your teeth fall out but the one that gives you a toothache for the rest of your life."

Of all curses, though, none is as evil as this one: "May your doctors find your illness interesting enough to describe it in a case report!"

Such was the misfortune of a 51-year-old surgeon, Dr. A, whose tale was described in The New England Journal of Medicine:

It was late on a summer day of fishing in coastal New England seawaters. Dr. A was cleaning the fish he had caught using a fillet knife when he noticed that he had accidentally cut the tip of his ring finger. 'Just a cut,' he thought, as he stopped the bleeding, applying direct pressure to the open, fresh wound.

But from that moment on, he was destined to face a series of unfortunate events.

Twelve hours after his injury, he awoke with throbbing pain in his fingertip. He took a dose of antibiotics. The pain, though, increased, and his finger became red. Dr. A's physician recognized the severity of the condition and walked him down the hall, immediately, to a hand surgeon.

Over the next several hours, Dr. A's condition continued to deteriorate. His temperature spiked to 100.5° Fahrenheit. He could no longer move his ring finger. It was tender to the touch and swollen. It looked like an uncooked sausage. It felt even worse.

Quickly thereafter, Dr. A's fever went up to 101.3. He became sluggish and apathetic. A blood test showed that the number of white blood cells – the army of cells specializing in fighting infections – was elevated. It became clear that Dr. A's condition was serious, that his body was trying, in vain, to fight a devastating infection, and that without urgent intervention, his condition could further deteriorate.

Before I proceed with this story, there is something I need to tell you about the hand. It is a highly complex, fascinating structure that serves a function: to grasp and release, play and create, manipulate and translate ideas of movement into actual movement. The hand has 27 bones and 34 muscles which move the fingers and thumb, 18 of which are in the forearm. It is innervated by three nerves and supplied by two main blood vessels. These structures are divided into several distinct compartments. Each compartment is a closed system wrapped in an envelope of connective tissue.

Now, back to Dr. A's story: His injury was not "just a cut," but a port of entry for bacteria to invade his body, his kingdom. His immune system sensed the danger. His white blood cells, the soldiers of the kingdom, were quickly called into action. They formed in large groups and moved quickly, mobilizing forces along the highways, within the blood vessels, searching everywhere for the enemy. All the while, though, the bacteria were moving upward along Dr. A's arm, along the compartment which they entered. They weren't moving along the highways. Instead, they were advancing through the "underground channels" in the small gaps between Dr. A's muscles and the envelopes around them, practically invisible to the antibiotics and the immune soldiers of A's body.

It was time to expose the invaders. Dr. A and his immune system could not do that alone. It was time to take to the knife – a time for a hand surgeon, and his scalpel.

In the operating room, lights on, wrapped in scrubs, and ready for action, Dr. A's doctors noticed a long streak of redness extending from the tip of his finger all the way to his underarm. Ominous, dark clouds quickly descended upon them, and sweat broke out on their upper lips, under their surgical masks. Were the bacteria moving along Dr. A's arm? Were they spreading the way bacteria sometimes do in the upper extremity: first by gaining entry through a cut, then by moving along the "underground channels," escaping the molecules of antibiotics, invisible to the immune cells, the soldiers of Dr. A's kingdom?

The doctors cut into the skin and deep into the sheath that surrounds the muscles and tendons in the infected finger. They saw cloudy fluid slowly oozing from the wound. They washed the wound with copious amounts of salt water. They left it open to allow the infection to drain, to air, to clean itself from the inside out. They prescribed antibiotics that would cover all imaginable bacteria: bacteria living in seawater, bacteria dwelling on fish, and resistant bacteria that colonize health care providers such as Dr. A.

On the next day, during evening rounds, Dr. A's temperature continued to rise. He lost sensation in his ring finger. His ring finger became necrotic (Medicalese for: it was still attached, but literally dead).

Back in the O.R., the doctors removed the necrotic finger and opened the sheath that surrounds the muscles and tendons of the ring finger in the hand and along the forearm. They extended the antibiotics coverage.

The following morning (the fourth day after the injury), the pain continued. The doctors performed more surgery: more irrigations and deeper cuts into the sheathes of the hand and the arm.

Agony. Fear. Horror.

When a wound heals, when a patient is cured, both the doctor and the patient laugh together. When wounds refuse to heal, when a cure is out of reach, when hope dissipates, when the realization of finality sinks in, the patient cries, and his doctor cries too.

And that, I believe, is what happened to Dr. A and his doctors. Later that day, the fever kept spiking, the pain worsened, and the doctors gathered. They looked at their patient, who was a doctor, one of their own, a surgeon whose livelihood was dependent on his manual dexterity. They knew what needed to be done. They took him back to the operating room and amputated his forearm. Doctors call it "guillotine amputation," for it is as pleasant as the French Revolution.

Over the next several days, A's condition improved. The fever abated, and there was no sign of infection. Six months later, The New England Journal of Medicine reported, "he was fitted with a prosthetic limb and returned to his clinical practice in a modified role."

I told you that of all curses, none is as evil as this one: "may your doctors find your illness interesting enough to describe it in a case report." The case of Dr. A proves my point. But there is a silver lining to stories like Dr. A's story: A case report is a medical tale of the extraordinary. It is an *exception* that proves the rule – of miraculous immune response, and of complete healing. In almost all cases, a cut is, well, just a cut.

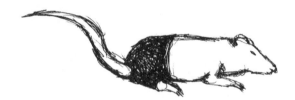

RATS IN PANTS

Urologists are a curious, creative bunch. And a curious mind often stumbles upon ideas never before conceived. I will tell you three short stories, all of them true, about urologists and their extraordinary ideas. Two of these urologists won the Nobel Prize in Physiology and Medicine for their achievements. The third won the Ig Nobel prize – a parody of the Nobel prize given out for unusual or trivial scientific achievements "that first make people laugh, and then make them think."

Werner Theodore Otto Forssmann was born in Berlin, in 1904. In 1929 he became a doctor. Forssmann wanted to be an internist, but his application was rejected. He tried Gynecology, but after "three miserable weeks in midwifery," he accepted a different position in a rural hospital in the Department of Surgery.

Once there, the young Dr. Forssmann asked his mentor, Dr. Richard Schneider, for permission to self-experiment with cardiac catheterization: he wanted to pass a small-caliber tube (a catheter) through a vein in his forearm into his heart. Forssmann believed that such a procedure, if proved possible, would allow delivery of lifesaving medications directly into the heart. To prove his point, he was willing to perform the experiment on himself.

Dr. Schneider, a logical, cautious man, swiftly rejected the very dangerous idea. The enthusiastic and intrepid Forssmann was not deterred. His first experiment was discontinued prematurely, for the surgical colleague who was passing the catheter through Forssmann's vein suddenly lost courage and refused to pass the catheter all the way into Forssmann's heart.

Forssmann then asked Gerda Ditzen, a nurse that was working with him, for help. She agreed to provide the necessary surgical instruments, but insisted that *she* would be the first subject of the experiment.

Forssmann played along. He strapped the nurse to the operating table in preparation for surgery. He prepared the incision site on her arm with iodine, perhaps even gave her local anesthesia. But then, he turned away from her and while she was tied down, unable to prevent him from carrying out his plan, he performed the procedure on himself, passing the catheter all the way, for a length of 65 centimeters, into his heart.

When she recognized the deceit, Ditzen became angry, but then, she quickly resumed her role as a nurse, helping Forssmann walk down the corridors and downstairs – with the catheter still in his heart – to the X-ray suite where an X-ray study confirmed that the catheter was indeed in Forssmann's heart.

The results of his experiments, published in 1929, were met with skepticism, controversy, hostility, and turmoil. Professor Ferdinand Sauerbruch said: "With work like this you qualify in a circus, but not in a reputable clinic."

Forssmann continued to experiment with cardiac catheterization, a total of nine self-experiments. He was discouraged, though, by the treatment of his peers, and so, when the opportunity arose, he accepted a position as a urologist in the only department specializing in urology in Berlin at the time. He continued to publish scientific articles, but his emphasis shifted from the heart to the prostate, bladder, and kidneys. He became a urologist.

In 1956, Forssmann was awarded the Nobel Prize, along with Andre Cournard and Dickinson W. Richards, for "discoveries concerning heart catheterization and the pathologic changes in the circulatory system."

Forssmann never returned to the field of cardiology. "... When I considered it objectively I was certain I'd never be able to catch up ..." he said.

Today, cardiac catheterization is performed for both diagnostic and therapeutic reasons. A small catheter is introduced into a blood vessel that leads to the heart. The pressures and blood flow within the heart can be measured. Contrast dye can be injected through the catheter while X-rays are taken, allowing delineation of the arteries supplying the heart (coronary arteries). If a blockage in a coronary artery is identified, the blockage can be cleared and a stent (a tiny metal tubular scaffold) can be left in the artery to keep it open. More than a million cardiac catheterizations are performed each year in the US.

Werner Theodore Otto Forssmann, a doctor, a man who ended up being a urologist, had changed the field of cardiology.

Even if you listen carefully, you cannot hear your cells talking. But they do; they converse and instruct each other. Their voice is carried not by sound waves, but by molecules called hormones. This is a story about a urologist, Charles Brenton Huggins, who not only listened to the conversation between cells, but also chimed in, and by doing so, was able to extend the lives of millions of cancer patients.

Dr. Huggins, a Canadian-born doctor, did not plan on being a urologist. After obtaining a medical degree from Harvard University, he was originally slated to perform thyroid surgery at the Billings Hospital at the University of Chicago. When the need arose, though, for someone to perform cystoscopies (in which a small camera is used to examine the inside of the bladder), he obliged, later to become a leader in the field of urology. As a researcher, his main interest lay in both urological and cancer research.

Dr. Huggins knew that cells talk to each other, and that they do so, among other ways, by using hormones. Cells in the pituitary gland, a pea-size gland at the base of the brain, for example, make a hormone called Luteinizing hormone, then release it into the blood stream. Luteinizing hormone tells cells in the testicles to produce testosterone. The cells within the testicles oblige, and testosterone is made and released into the bloodstream. Testosterone, in turn, instructs different cell groups in different tissues and organs to change. During puberty in boys, for example, testosterone encourages tissues within the testicles and penis to enlarge, and pubic hair follicles to suddenly grow hair. The voice begins to deepen. Muscle cells grow. Sex drive develops. Testosterone calls on almost each and every cell in a boy's body to change, and so turns boys into men.

Dr. Huggins knew that pre-pubertal castration (and thus the elimination of testosterone production) had multiple effects on the body, including inhibition of prostate growth. In a series of experiments in dogs, Huggins demonstrated that male sex hormones stimulated the function and growth of the dogs' prostates, whereas female sex hormones inhibited them.

Are the effects of hormones limited to normal cells? Do cancer cells also "listen" to hormonal messages? And if so, could a change in the hormonal environment halt the proliferation of cancer cells, even kill them?

Dr. Huggins decided to experiment on a group of men with advanced prostate cancer. Some of these patients had cancer that had spread to their bones.

I can only imagine the doctor-patient conversations that took place, the explanations that were given to these unfortunate cancer patients about prostate cancer and testosterone, and how changing their hormonal environment might help them to combat cancer. "I am requesting your permission to eliminate the source of testosterone in your body by removing both of your testicles," Dr. Huggins must have told his patients. Asked if he had ever tried it before, he must have responded with a resounding "No."

This was the early 1940s, and no other treatment for advanced prostate cancer was available. And so, whether it was out of trust in Dr. Huggins and his ideas, or out of sheer despair, some patients agreed to participate in the study. They were treated with either exogenous estrogen (a female hormone), or with bilateral orchiectomy (surgical castration, or removal of both testicles).

The results were astonishing. Dr. Huggins discovered that the hormonal treatments he designed did lead to a decrease in the activity of prostate cancer cells. And a significant subset of patients responded well: Their primary tumor shrank, their bone pain subsided, they regained some of the weight they had lost fighting their cancer, and four of the 24 patients lived for more than a decade after their treatment.

For these discoveries, Dr. Huggins received the Nobel Prize. In the presentation speech for the Nobel Prize, Professor G. Klein said: "These patients who would not have had more than a short time to live without this treatment, frequently became free of symptoms for many years..."

Dr. Huggins brought to the forefront the idea that some types of cancer cells are dependent on hormones, and that altering their hormonal environment may lead to the death of cancer cells. A new type of cancer treatment has since evolved, and is still in use today in the treatment of both prostate cancer and breast cancer.

Upon receiving the Nobel Prize for his discovery, Charles Huggins said, with humility: "A cancer worker utters the mariner's prayer: 'Oh, Lord, Thy sea is so vast and my bark is so small.'"

The Ig Nobel prize, a parody of the Nobel prize, is given out for unusual or trivial scientific achievements "that first make people laugh, and then make them think."

The 2016 Ig Nobel Prize was awarded to the late Professor Ahmed Shafik, an Egyptian urologist from Cairo University in Egypt. He was a prolific researcher who published more than 1000 articles in the medical literature.

Here is what you need to know about the study that won Professor Shafik the Ig Nobel Prize:

For the purpose of this study, small pants were designed to fit over the the lower body of rats. The pants would cover their lower back, their scrotal and penile areas, and the upper parts of their lower limbs. Small openings were made for the anal orifice, penis, and tail. The pants were fastened to the rats' bodies with a small string at their waist.

Seventy-five rats participated in the study. They were divided into 5 equal groups (15 rats in each). Four of the groups were dressed in textile pants, made of either 100% polyester, 100% cotton, 50% polyester/50% cotton mix, or 100% wool. The fifth group, which served as a control group, remained *au naturel*.

The rats in this study fared much better than the average lab rat. They were not probed, force-fed, or sacrificed at the end of the study. Instead, they were housed two per cage and received the standard rat chow and bedding. They were allowed to copulate whenever their hearts desired. In an illustration that accompanied the article describing the results of Dr. Shafik's study, one particular rat is shown modeling its pants. It looks quite content.

Shafik wanted to know what effect different types of textile have on sexual activity. He assessed the sexual behavior of the different groups before the pants were applied, after 6 and 12 months of wearing the pants, and 6 months after the pants were removed. He found that after 6 and 12 months, the rate of intromission (penetration) in the groups wearing the polyester and polyester/cotton mix was lower than in the pre-test levels and lower than in the other groups (cotton, wool, and naked). The reduction in the rate of intromission was more pronounced in the 100% polyester group. The reduction in the rate of intromission was also more pronounced after 12 months than after 6 months.

Dr. Shafik concluded that rats in polyester pants experience a decrease in their sexual activity. But why? To answer this question, Shafik measured the electrostatic potentials generated on the penis and scrotum. He discovered that the polyester pants generated electrostatic potentials, whereas the other textiles did not. Shafik attributed the change in the rats' sexual behavior to the electrostatic fields generated by the polyester fabric.

On September 3, 2016, the Ig Nobel Prizes were awarded in a ceremony at Harvard's Sanders Theatre. The Reproduction Prize went posthumously to Dr. Shafik. Other winners in economics, physics, chemistry, psychology, and other fields were also announced. The Ig Nobel prize in medicine went to Christoph Helmchen and his collaborators for discovering that "if you have an itch on the left side of your body, you can relieve it by looking in the mirror and scratching the right side of your body (and vice versa)."

Dr. Shafik's study made me laugh, then think. I looked out my window and imagined myself standing outside in an upper peninsula blizzard wearing boots, waterproof pants, a heavy coat, gloves, and a Stormy Kromer. I imagined myself as a baker wearing red silicone mitts, pulling steamy, hot loaves of bread out of the oven. I imagined myself as a knight in armor. I thought about the different ways clothing protects us. I thought about the constant game of hide and seek we play, using clothing to conceal parts of our bodies and to reveal others, to show off and attract, and, at times, to just blend in a crowd.

But mostly, I thought about clothing as an expression, a statement of who we are and what we represent: as individuals, as members of our cultural group, as professionals. I remembered myself attending medical meetings mummified in a three-piece blue suit, a tight collar shirt, and a tie to match; and in the operating room wearing itchy, green, polyester scrubs. What is the price we pay, I ask myself, in terms of comfort, for dressing up to code? And what is the price we pay in terms of our own health?

Nowadays, if you come to see me in my office, you will find me in light pants, a comfortable shirt, and a long white coat, all made of 100% cotton. And I am as content as the rat in Dr. Shafik's illustration, a rat in 100% cotton pants.

A SALTY PATIENT

Patients called her Dr. Tamara. She did look like a doctor: she wore a white coat, she had a stethoscope hanging around her neck, and she seemed busy all the time, as if she were rushing to save the life of yet another patient. Yet she was still only a medical student. And she had deep doubts in her heart about whether she should even become a doctor, whether she could ever be a good doctor.

Tamara had doubts about whether she should become a doctor because when she applied for medical school, her father had told her that the doctors he knew were all sad people. "Doctors witness pain. They encounter great suffering. Doctors fight the inevitable," he said, and added, "think engineering instead." And Eli, her fiancé of three years, told her, just weeks after she had entered medical school, that she had no time or energy for him anymore. "It's not me, it's you," he said. "You married Medicine and divorced me, and left the real world altogether." A couple of weeks after he left her, she saw him on Bugrashov street, holding hands with Rachel, who was taller than her, blonder, wore no glasses, and did not have a lazy eye.

Tamara envied doctors like Dr. Solomon, who seemed to have not even a shred of doubt. Dr. Solomon did not look like a typical doctor. He had red, wild, curly hair. He wore a wrinkled white coat, a stethoscope that was always on the verge of falling out of his pocket, unmatched socks, and sandals. Sitting amongst her fellow medical students, around a large oval desk in the conference room attached to the Med/Surg floor, Dr. Solomon told the group that he would be their instructor on the Internal Medicine rotation for the next few weeks. He did not seem to be overly excited about it.

"This is 'Harrison's Principles of Internal Medicine', our textbook," Dr. Solomon said as he carefully placed the book on the desk. The book was thick, the pages were as thin as garlic skin, the fonts were small – between its covers, Harrison's carried an insurmountable amount of medical knowledge. "And here is a needle," Dr. Solomon continued, as he pulled a needle from his worn leather briefcase. He then turned to Tamara who sat next to him. "To prove that I know this book by heart," Dr. Solomon announced, as if he were a magician preparing to cut a woman in half, "I will ask Tamara to point the tip of the needle at any random point on the book cover, and I will ask you to imagine her piercing through the book with the needle. I will then tell you to pick a number, any page number you wish, and I will tell you the exact word, the subject matter, and the chapter that the needle would poke through on that page. Just pick a page number, would you?"

Tamara held the needle perpendicular to the book and aimed it at a point in the upper left side of Harrison's. "Which word would appear on page 373?" she asked. Dr. Solomon closed his eyes and concentrated. "The chapter is 'Infections of the Upper Respiratory Systems' and the word is 'voluntary.' He could then tell what words and which chapters were on pages 875, 1596, and 2743. Tamara swiftly concluded that the man was a genius.

Throughout the Internal Medicine rotation, Dr. Solomon continued to teach Tamara and the other students by using playful games, by presenting them with curious riddles. He took Tamara and her fellow students on "field trips" around the hospital. He told them that in order to make the right diagnosis, a good doctor should use all five, even six senses. "Today," Dr. Solomon said quietly, as he leaned against the wall of the hospital lobby, "we will focus on vision. Look at the patients and the visitors who are passing by and make a diagnosis using the power of observation alone. Observe their eyes, their face, their hands, their posture, their gait. I will take the first turn."

The group of students followed Dr. Solomon as he

walked, scanning the crowd of patients, visitors, nurses, and doctors. Standing next to the elevators, he found an elderly patient wearing a hospital gown who seemed pleasantly confused, and also happy to participate in his "diagnosis by observation" game. Dr. Solomon pointed at a small, yellow deposition of fat close to the man's upper eyelid. "Xanthelasma," he said. "It is a sign of high cholesterol levels. Now it is your turn. Make a diagnosis."

Minutes later, Tamara offered her own diagnosis of a middle-aged woman whose fingers were bent. "Swan-neck deformity," Tamara said proudly, "a sign of rheumatoid arthritis." Dr. Solomon nodded.

Each day, as they were taking a lunch break between lectures, Dr. Solomon encouraged his students to create lists. "Name and briefly discuss diseases that begin with the letter X." Or, "make a list of diseases that can be diagnosed using only your stethoscope." Toward the end of their rotation, Dr. Solomon asked the group to make a list of devastating diseases caused by a small defect in a single protein, and another list of medical conditions that can be diagnosed by using the sense of taste. These two lists were never discussed in class.

The rotation in Internal Medicine was coming to an end, and all that was left was the final test. "For the final exam," Dr. Solomon told the group, "imagine yourself on a lonely island with three patients whose lives depend on you making the correct diagnosis. It is nighttime, and you are the only doctor available on the island. Modern technology has not yet reached your lonely island. There are no laboratories and no test results, no radiology department and no imaging studies. It is you and these three souls whose lives depend on you. It is time for you to practice what we have learned in class. To make a diagnosis, a correct one, using your senses alone."

Dr. Tamara doubted whether she could pass the final exam.

On a hot summer day, the last day of the Internal Medicine rotation, Dr. Tamara's mission was to correctly diagnose three different patients in three different rooms. Yes, she felt that the elderly man, who was short of breath and had swollen ankles, had congestive heart failure. And that the middle-aged woman with a small constricted mouth, who complained that her fingers turned blue in the cold, was a victim of her own immune system and had scleroderma. But the man waiting for her in the third examination room seemed too young to belong in the Internal Medicine department. Actually, Tamara thought, he was too young to be sick. Still, he was there, accompanied by his mother. He was the last of the three patients whose medical puzzle she needed to solve.

"My name is Dan," he told her, after she had introduced herself, thanking him for volunteering to be a patient on her test. Dan was 19 year old. He was thin, too thin.

His eyes were sad, but curious. He had a kind smile. Tamara could see that Dan was short of breath. Shaking his hands, Tamara noticed that his fingers were thickened at the ends, like drumsticks, and that his fingernails were wide and round, like watch-glass.

They all played their parts. Tamara asked questions the way doctors do, and Dan and his mother told her his unfortunate tale of pain and sorrow, completing each other's sentences and nodding at each other's words the way people do when they tell a story for the thousandth time.

As far back as they could remember, Dan was always coughing and short of breath. He was shorter than other children his age and slimmer, despite having an excellent appetite. "It is embarrassing to say, but I think it is important for you to know," his mother said, "for your test, I mean, that his bowel movements are bulky, greasy, and smelly too. And that he has had many bouts of pneumonia like the one he has now."

"Will it be okay if I examine you?" Tamara asked Dan. She palpated his neck for enlarged lymph nodes and examined his clubbed fingers. She turned off the air conditioner, which made more noise than cool air, and pulled out her Littmann stethoscope. She closed her eyes and carefully listened to Dan's pounding heart, and to his wheezing lungs. "Take a deep breath and hold," she asked. Dan started coughing again.

Tamara took a step back and made a few notes in her

pocket book. "So, can you figure out what is wrong with me?" he asked her, a smile on his face, "I can give you a hint."

"You are very kind, Dan," she smiled back at him, "but no hints are allowed. How about we play a 'hot and cold' game? I will tell you a story about you and your cells, and you will tell me if I am getting closer to making the correct diagnosis."

Dan and his mother loved the idea.

"Your body is made of billions of cells," she told Dan. "Each cell produces about 20,000 proteins. Some of these proteins are critical for individual cells to carry out a specific task. What if one of these proteins is defective?"

"Hot," Dan said.

"This defective protein that I am talking about," Tamara continued, "plays a role in different cells in different parts of your body. A defective protein in the lungs will make the mucous in the lung thicker and more difficult to clear. You will therefore suffer from thick sputum, constant coughing, and chronic lung infections."

Dan and his mother nodded.

"And in the digestive system, the same defective protein will cause the fluids produced in the pancreas to be thicker, making proper digestion nearly impossible. You will end up with bulky, greasy, bowel movements."

"Very hot. You are getting much closer," Dan said.

At this point, Tamara was almost sure that she had arrived at the correct diagnosis. In her mind, Tamara could hear Dr. Solomon's voice: "Make a list of devastating diseases caused by a small defect in a single protein and another list of diseases that can be diagnosed by using your sense of taste." She could hear him say: "It is time for you to practice what we have learned in class and to make a diagnosis, a correct one, using your senses alone." Dr. Solomon was not just dropping hints – he was giving her the correct answer!

"So," Dan asked, "do you know what the correct diagnosis is?"

"Can I taste your sweat?" Tamara asked.

This proposition would sound curious in any other circumstance and perhaps more so in a meeting between a patient and a doctor, but it seemed natural to Tamara and Dan, for they knew that she was as close to making the absolutely, positively correct diagnosis as one can be ("Burning hot! BURNING HOT!" he said, as he agreed). They knew that the same defective protein that wreaked havoc in Dan's lungs and intestines could also cause a change in the chemical composition of his sweat.

Tamara passed her finger along the side of Dan's forehead and then brought her finger to her mouth. Dan's sweat was salty, very salty.

"Cystic fibrosis," she told Dan. "That is my final diagnosis."

"Bingo!" he replied.

On that hot summer day, in the moments that followed her final exam, Tamara had no more doubts about whether she could become the good doctor she so desired to be. She realized that she could interlace signs and symptoms, threads of welt and warp, and weave them into a precise story of patient and disease.

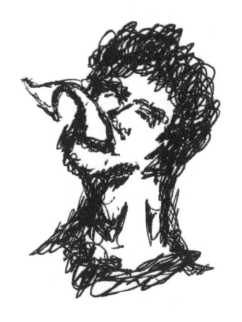

THE MAN WHO SWALLOWED A FISH

It was a cold winter day in Akron, Ohio. Mr. Gentner, a 23-year-old man, choked to death after trying to swallow a live, 5-inch-long fish. According to the New York Times, the three friends who dared the man to swallow the fish called 911, reporting that Mr. Gentner had a fish stuck in his throat and that he was having trouble breathing. The paramedics could see the tail still sticking out of his mouth, but they could not resuscitate him.

Later, Mr. Gentner was awarded a Darwin Award, an honor bestowed upon individuals who, according to the Darwin Awards website, "protect our gene pool by making the ultimate sacrifice of their own lives," and "eliminate themselves in an extraordinarily idiotic manner, thereby improving our species' chances of long-term survival."

The list of Darwin Awards winners is long – and curious.

Researchers from the Institute of Cellular Medicine, Newcastle University, United Kingdom, reviewed the data on Darwin Awards winners between 1995 and 2014, a 20-year period. Their goal was to examine sex differences in idiotic risk-taking behavior. They found that men are significantly more likely to win the award: of the 332 cases verified and confirmed by the Darwin Awards Committee, only "14 were shared by male and female nominees—usually overly adventurous couples in compromising positions." Of the 318 remaining cases, 282 Darwin Awards were awarded to men and only 36 awards were given to women.

From a statistical standpoint, the difference in idiotic risk-taking behavior between men and women was significant: men made up 88.7% of the Darwin Awards winners. From a man's standpoint, the difference is worrisome, astonishing, perhaps even one that may provoke self-reflection. From a woman's standpoint, I imagine the response to be expressed in a single, coherent sentence: "I told you so!"

Why are men more likely to win a Darwin Award? One explanation, the authors suggest, is consistent with the male-idiot-theory (or MIT, in short), proclaiming that "men are idiots and idiots do stupid things." This, to me, sounds awfully sexist.

Another explanation points to the fact that some of

the winners found their death while intoxicated. It is not inconceivable to assume that men drink more alcohol than women and that excessive alcohol consumption may impair judgement—"alcohol makes men feel 'bullet-proof' after a few drinks," the authors suggest. And feeling bullet-proof does not necessarily make you immortal.

Other scientists may claim that the study is a retrospective one and therefore may carry significant bias. Conspiracy theorists may go even further, suggesting that the results may be intentionally biased: It is possible, they might claim, that women nominate more men for the award, or that the Darwin Awards committee is, for one reason or another, biased towards selecting more men.

Societal influence, rather than lack of self-reflection and good judgment, may also be a factor contributing to the overwhelmingly macho nature of idiotic death: call it a rite of passage, pursuit of societal esteem, or just an attempt to earn bragging rights, these poor men may be the victims of a society that is pushing some of its members to illogical, absurd, even deadly behavior.

Is idiotic risk-taking behavior a selection process whereby individuals selflessly remove themselves from the gene pool, allowing others a selective advantage?

The theory, most probably untrue and definitely unproven, is entertaining to the authors and to many readers. In response to the article, Robert Sirota from Hundingdon Valley, Pa., writes: "The article is a bright spot in an otherwise dreary and depressing world. I did not take it seriously, and I do not think anyone else should. It was funny, and there is not much difference between it and stand-up humor."

The article was published in the British Medical Journal, one of the most prestigious medical journals (it is ranked fifth, according to its impact factor, among general medical journals). It was, however, a part of the BMJ's Christmas issue, which takes a humorous, "goofy" approach and publishes articles examining profound medical dilemmas, such as how much James Bond actually drank, and why Rudolph's nose was red.

Christopher W. Benson, a Pathology Analyst from Cardiff, UK, disagrees. He writes: "This is a joke article but the joke is not funny... Perhaps it would have been funnier if your source data had not been obtained from a list of, however idiotic, tragic deaths of real people."

And I think: the good humorist puts a mirror in front of us. We look closely and see ourselves—a reflection of the village idiot, or the Darwin Awards winner. We laugh, we cry, we learn.

ALBERT'S PAIN

On a cloudy Tuesday evening, in the fall of 2016, Albert's life was about to become even more complicated.

Albert was 32. His dog, Blacky, had died several weeks earlier. He and his girlfriend Georgina had just moved into a small rental apartment. Albert and Georgina's belongings, still in boxes, were scattered all over the floor of the living room, their bed, and their kitchen table. The neighbor downstairs, a retired teacher who wore glasses so thick you could never see his eyes, practiced drumming when he felt lonely every night.

Albert had just started a new job as a sales manager in a downtown store selling recliners, the brand name of which rhymed with 'Hazy Toy.' When Albert took the job, he was told that the recliners just sell themselves.

That wasn't true. Some customers raised concerns about the stain-resistance qualities of the fabric, others were questioning the durability of the electrical reclining mechanism; the cushions were not soft enough, and besides, the recliners were too expensive. Albert's base salary was small, and he never earned a bonus.

Tuesdays were particularly slow. On his way home from work, Albert bought a large pepperoni pizza and a six-pack of beer. Georgina was away, visiting her sister. Albert was resting in the living room and binge-watching Breaking Bad. He was eating his pizza, one slice after another, and drinking beer, one can after another. Downstairs, Eyeglasses was drumming a tune that sounded almost like Ain't Misbehavin'.

An hour later (the pizza box was empty, the beer cans were rolling on the floor), Albert suddenly felt a "crushing pain" in his chest. He was short of breath, and nauseated. He was sweating all over. He went to the bathroom and stuck two fingers in his mouth, trying to throw up, but nothing came out. He found TUMS tablets in one of the boxes and took two, but the pain only intensified. Albert called 911 and was taken by an ambulance to the emergency room.

The ER doctor asked Albert about his pain, the way many good doctors do, by following the PQRST mnemonic:

P stands for provocation and palliation: what makes the pain worse, what makes it better?

Q for quality: is the pain sharp or dull? Is it stabbing, burning, or crushing?

R for radiation: where did the pain start? Does it radiate anywhere else? Did it start elsewhere and then move to its current location?

S for severity: how intense is the pain on a scale of 1-10?

T for time: when did the pain start, and how long did it last?

Here is a short story about the PQRST mnemonic and chest pain. The story is taken from my medical school days: Sackler School of Medicine was a 10-floor building with three main elevators. Eliezer Kaplinski, a professor of cardiology, was our teacher. His hair was always well-kept, and his stethoscope was always slightly protruding from the inner pocket of his 3-piece suit. We listened very carefully in Kaplinski's class and wrote down every word of wisdom he uttered, because we knew that in the final exam, Kaplinski would not use questions written by a teaching assistant, or taken from a database of pre-written questions. Instead, Kaplinski himself would write the questions and make them complex enough to challenge even the brightest of students. So, it comes as no surprise that I remember Kaplinski's words about diagnosing heart attacks using the PQRST mnemonic: "a classic heart attack is an elevator diagnosis," he said. "Enter the elevator with a patient on the ground floor, ask him the right questions about his chest pain, and when you reach the tenth floor, you should have made the correct diagnosis."

Kaplinski taught us that the typical warning sign of a heart attack is chest pain that feels like uncomfortable pressure, squeezing, or fullness; that the pain typically lasts for a few minutes and may radiate to one or both arms, the back, neck, jaw or stomach. He told us that shortness of breath may accompany the chest pain, and that other symptoms may include cold sweats, nausea, and light-headedness.

Back to Albert in the emergency room: when asked where his pain was, Albert pointed to his xiphoid (the lowest part of his sternum, or chest-bone). He told the doctor that the pain started after he ate a whole pizza and drank a six-pack of beer, and that he had been under a lot of stress at work; he told the doctor that the pain was 7 out of 10 in severity, and that it radiated nowhere. "It started about two hours ago and it is still going," he said, and then added, "it is a crushing pain." Albert also told the doctor that his father had acute chest pain at a young age, and was later diagnosed with heart disease.

The doctor pressed his stethoscope to Albert's chest and closed his eyes. The heart rate was normal, and there were no murmurs, he noticed. An electrocardiogram showed only subtle changes in the electrical activity of Albert's heart. This could be consistent with a heart attack, the doctor thought, or not. A lab technician took a blood sample, but there was no time to wait for the results. Listening to Albert's story and to how he described his pain, the doctor thought that a heart attack was a likely diagnosis. And because a heart attack can kill, he gave Albert Aspirin, heparin, and nitroglycerin, and ordered some more tests.

Here is something I wanted to tell you about pain: People who believe that there is order in the universe, that there is purpose in nature, would tell you that pain is a warning sign – like a red light flashing on your dashboard indicating that you are running out of gas, your oil is low, your engine needs service, or that you need to wear a seatbelt.

In Albert's case, the blood test for cardiac enzymes, which are often elevated in patients with a heart attack, came back normal. And an emergency coronary angiography – an X-ray test that checks if the arteries supplying the heart are open – showed no blockage and a good, functioning heart. The red flashing light on Albert's dashboard was signaling a heart attack, but a heart attack it was not.

It was time to consider other possible causes of Albert's chest pain. Doctors call this "differential diagnosis." They consider all possible causes for pain. They narrow down the number of potential diagnoses by obtaining more information. They systematically rule out unlikely diagnoses. And then they reach a final, hopefully correct diagnosis.

In the case of chest pain, the list of potential diagnoses is long and ominous. And in some patients, chest pain is a symptom of a disease that originates elsewhere: a gastric ulcer, biliary colic, or herpes zoster.

After his angiography, Albert told his doctors that the pain in his chest had shifted to his right upper abdomen. Several hours later, the color in his eyes turned yellow, and his urine became dark. His blood test showed high bilirubin levels and an ultrasound examination confirmed that there was a stone in his gallbladder. These were all indications that he might have acute cholecystitis (inflammation of the gallbladder), or that he might have passed a gallbladder stone.

To prevent future gallstone episodes, Albert's doctors decided to surgically remove his gallbladder. During surgery, they found a very distended, severely inflamed gallbladder, with a necrotic wall that was threatening to burst. The pathologist told them later that within the gallbladder, he found a large number of irregular, roughly spherical, yellow and yellowish-green gallbladder stones.

About the true nature of pain, I will tell you this: pain is not the best of alarm systems, and it doesn't always work as well as the flashing red lights on the dashboard of your car. The body's pain mechanism suffers from the following shortcomings:

The body's pain mechanism isn't reliable: the red light signal might start flashing for no good reason (an intense headache may make you feel like you are going to die, but such headaches are only rarely caused by brain tumors).

The body pain mechanism is disproportionate — there is poor correlation between the intensity of the signal and the severity of the underlying condition. In other words, the red light signal might be flashing hysterically when the windshield fluid is half full, but it flashes only occasionally, and faintly, when the brakes are failing (a kidney stone which is a benign, highly treatable condition, could give you the worst pain of your life; cancer is often painless until it is too late to cure).

The body pain mechanism has poor specificity: the red light might start flashing for the wrong reason (you didn't wear your seatbelt, but it tells you that your oil runs low, or, as in Albert's case, a chest pain indicates a gallbladder disease, not a heart attack.)

Pain isn't the ideal alarm system, but it is the best we have. It should not be ignored, for in many cases, pain is a symptom of a significant medical problem, sometimes urgent, that should be addressed.

As for Albert, three weeks after his surgery, his chest pain was gone. He was doing just fine.

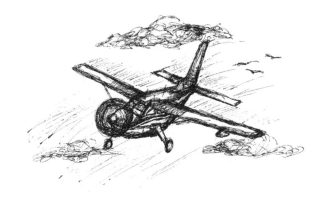

THE AVIATORS

The other day, Dr. C, a cardiologist, came up to me with a tempting proposition. It turns out that a friend of his, also a doctor, owns an airplane. "Do you want to buy my friend's plane?" he asked me. And then he added: "If you buy the aircraft – believe me when I tell you it is beautiful, white with red and blue stripes running along its sides, two wings and twin propeller engines – my friend will pay for your flying lessons, and it will be a lot of fun. To fly, I mean."

"I don't believe in doctors flying their own airplanes; they tend to crash," I said," and choosing between the fun of flying and the boredom of staying on the ground, alive, I would take the second option, time and time again."

To my surprise, and in a complete reversal of his initial proposal, yet still in a calm, quiet, measured voice, Dr. C was quick to wholeheartedly agree. He knew of at least one famous doctor, a cardiologist like himself, who died in an airplane crash: The famous cardiologist was Dr. Andreas Roland Gruentzig, a German cardiologist, a pioneer, a man who changed the field of Cardiology. In his kitchen, Gruentzig added an inflatable balloon to a small-caliber catheter. In September 1977, after improving on the prototype and experimenting on dogs and monkeys with his balloon-catheter, Gruentzig became the first doctor to perform a successful angioplasty on a wide-awake human being.

The patient, Adolph Bachman, was relatively young and otherwise healthy, but he had a severe obstruction (stenosis) in one of the main arteries supplying blood to his heart. Gruentzig gently navigated the catheter into the blocked segment, inflated the balloon, and using X-rays, watched the artery as it expanded, allowing blood to freely flow again. The patient's condition improved. His chest pain resolved. And ten years after the procedure, his coronary artery remained almost perfectly open.

Gruentzig's balloon catheter was a breakthrough. It was the first step in a revolution that would lead to the use of minimally-invasive procedures instead of more invasive open heart surgeries in many patients with blocked coronary arteries.

In 1985, Gruentzig and his wife died in an airplane accident during a rain storm. He was 46-year-old, and she was 29. He was the pilot in their Beechcraft-Baron airplane.

Listening to Dr. C's story about a cardiologist-aviator, I immediately responded with a story of my own about another doctor-aviator. The protagonist in my story was a renowned urologist, Dr. Brantley Scott, a professor of Urology at Baylor University College of Medicine. In the early 1970s, and almost 30 years before the development of Viagra, Scott contributed to the development of the inflatable penile prosthesis. The device includes two inflatable silicone cylinders that, once implanted into the corpora cavernosa of the penis, allows men with erectile dysfunction to obtain an erection. It has since been implanted in more than 100,000 men.

At the age of 61, and shortly after he announced his intention to retire, Scott died in an airplane accident. He was the pilot in a light Quest-Air single-engine plane which he had assembled himself from a kit.

"Interesting," said Dr. C, as he nodded. It was time for us to ponder on the frequent plane crashes among doctor-aviators: perhaps it was over-confidence – a sense of invulnerability that comes with the heroism of saving lives. Or mere inexperience, for a busy doctor could not fly as often as other pilots. "Could it be just bad luck?" he asked. "Perhaps we are just biased," he added, "because we know of more doctor-aviators than pilots in any other profession."

Whatever the explanation is, it became evident that I am not going to buy an airplane any time soon. We continued to talk about cardiology and urology, great medical innovators, and mutual patients. And just as we were about to part ways, Dr. C told me about another friend of his, a doctor, who owns a beautiful yacht. Then, he asked: "Perhaps you prefer to buy my friend's yacht?"

UNLUCKY STRIKE

Prince Leopold, the son of Queen Victoria, had suffered joint pain since he was young. At age 30, he followed his doctor's advice, kissed his pregnant wife Princess Helena goodbye, and travelled from the United Kingdom to his Cannes residence, the Villa Nevada, where the weather was supposed to be better for his joints. On March 27, 1884, while at the Villa, Prince Leopold slipped and fell. He injured his knee and his head. He died the next morning.

The fate of other descendants of Queen Victoria was as horrible as that of Prince Leopold. And since Queen Victoria's daughters married into the royal families of Germany, Spain, and Russia, it was a fate shared by several monarchies across Europe.

At age 2, Queen Victoria's grandson, Prince Friedrich of Hesse and by Rhine (German Empire) tumbled through a window and fell. He died several hours later of brain hemorrhage. Another grandson, Lord Leopold Mountbatten, died at age 32 during a hip operation.

Queen Victoria's great grandsons did not fare any better: At age 4, Prince Heinrich Friedrich of Prussia fell, head first, from a table and onto the floor. He died of a brain hemorrhage a few hours later. At age 20, as a result of a car accident, Prince Rupert of Teck died of intracerebral hemorrhage; at age 19, after a minor car accident (he was trying to avoid a cyclist), Infante Gonzalo of Spain died of severe abdominal bleeding; at age 31, Alfonso the Prince of Asturias crashed his car into a telephone booth. He sustained only minor injuries, but died of internal bleeding.

The astute reader (all of my readers are astute and possess a good sense of humor) must have noticed a pattern in the premature death habits of the royals: the royals died young, very young; they died of excessive bleeding; they died of injuries others might have survived; and they were all men.

Doctors and scientists have long suspected that the cause of the Royal Curse is hemophilia, a genetic disorder that impairs the body's ability to form blood clots. Patients with hemophilia bleed for longer periods of time even after minor injuries. When the bleeding occurs inside joints, it usually results in severe pain and joint damage. Some patients bleed during surgeries; others bleed into their brains, resulting in headaches, seizures, even death.

Was the Royal Disease indeed hemophilia?

It took several decades to answer this question with certainty. The answer lay in the story of another descendent of Queen Victoria – her great-grandson, Prince Alexei Romanov, who was the son of Tsar Nicholas II and heir to the Russian throne.

Here is his story. 1917 was a time of unrest and turmoil in Russia. World War I left Russia in worse shape than before: Millions of Russian men were taken away from their farms to join the war effort. 3,311,000 Russians lost their lives. Tzar Nicholas was blamed for the military defeats. Rumors had it that his wife, Tsarina Alexandra Feodorovna (who was a German), had tried to help Germany win the war. The price of food went up, and there were food shortages in the cities. Besides, it was winter – a cold, bitter, Russian winter. Laborers, peasants, serfs, and intellectuals weren't willing to tolerate the reign of the autocratic Tzar anymore. It was time for a revolution.

Thus, the Bolsheviks (the revolutionary troops) imprisoned Tsar Nicholas II, the Tsarina, and their five children in The House of Special Purpose where the royals were kept in strict isolation. The royals were no longer permitted to live like Tsars. The guards addressed them with contempt, by using only their names, not their titles. They had no access to their luggage; their money was confiscated; they had to part with their devoted servants, and to give up butter and coffee. They were constantly under surveillance. The house was protected by a fence and a tall palisade, four machine guns, and 300 guards. And the windows in all of the royal family's rooms were sealed shut and covered with newspapers.

On July 17, 1918, around midnight, the sleeping members of the royal family were awakened and ordered into the basement of the The House of Special Purpose. And the execution squad of the secret police was brought in. The neighbors heard multiple gunshots from afar. The basement was filled with the smell of gunpowder. The prince was shot several times, then stabbed, but somehow he was still alive. To complete the mission, Yakov Yurovsky, the commander of the secret police, shot the 13-year-old prince twice more, in the head. When the dust settled, when the cries of agony halted, all members of the Romanov royal family – Tsar Nicholas II, his wife, and their five children – were dead.

The remains (skeletal bones) of the two youngest members of the Romanov family, Prince Alexis and his sister, Anastasia, were not discovered until 2007.

Evgeny I. Rogaev, a researcher at the University of Massachusetts, and his colleagues carefully examined the remains of the Romanov family. They compared DNA extracted from the remains of the Romanov family to samples obtained from both maternal and paternal lineages of European royal families. They also compared the DNA to an archived 117-year-old blood specimen of Tsar Nicholas (when you are a Tsar, people tend to archive parts of your body, or just chop off your head). The researchers proved in an "accurate and unambiguous" way that the remains indeed belonged to the royal family.

Evgeny I. Rogaev went a step further. In a second article, published in the prestigious Science journal in 2009, he described how he and his collaborators applied genomic methods to sequence the DNA found in the remains of the royal family. This was not an easy task, because the amount of the DNA recovered was small and its quality was poor. Nevertheless, using sophisticated genomic processes, Evgeny overcame these obstacles. The researchers found a mutation located in the F9 (factor IX) gene, consistent with a severe form of hemophilia B called Christmas disease.

Hemophilia is caused by a mutation in the gene encoding for factor VIII (hemophilia A), or factor IX (hemophilia B). Factor VIII and IX are two of several factors (or proteins) essential to blood clotting. A mutation in the gene (DNA) encoding for these factors can result in severely decreased amounts of these clotting factors. As a result, blood does not clot, and bleedings do not stop.

The history of the royal family illustrates how hemophilia and similar diseases are transmitted. Scientists call this form of genetic transmission "X-linked," because it is caused by a mutation in the X chromosome. Here is how it happened:

Humans normally have 23 pairs of chromosomes, including one pair of sex chromosomes: XX in women, and XY in men.

Queen Victoria was born with the typical 23 pairs of chromosomes. However, a mutation had occurred in the DNA of one of her two X chromosomes. She had one normal X chromosome and one defective X chromosome. Her gametes (eggs) contained either one or the other.

Queen Victoria's daughters (XX) received one X chromosome from their father and one X chromosome from their mother. They were not affected by hemophilia, because the one normal X chromosome from their father was sufficient to encode for enough of the clotting factor. But they had a 50% chance to inherit a defective X chromosome from the queen, thus becoming a carrier of the disease.

Queen Victoria's male descendants (XY), on the other hand, received their Y chromosome from their father. They had a 50% chance of receiving a normal X chromosome and a 50% chance of receiving a defective X chromosome from their mother. And without a second, normal X chromosome to counterbalance the defective one, these royal descendants were doomed to suffer from the disease.

At times, one's fate is determined not by one's behavior, not by societal or historical circumstances, nor by the unique combination of normal genes inherited from his or her parents, but by a mutation that took place generations before – a single stroke of bad luck.

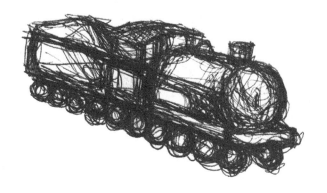

THREE TRAIN-RIDE TALES

A good train-ride story is always a tale of transformation. A passenger may find comfort in the pre-determined course, the well-grounded tracks, the monotonous rumbling sounds, and the gentle vibrations of the car. He may start a conversation with a fellow passenger, or just fall asleep. "It feels as if I have escaped time and place," he may tell himself, for every moment is as elusive as the scenery he sees through the windows. And as he moves through time, he is neither here nor there. Yet, in a good train-ride tale, the protagonist arriving at his destination is a man changed forever.

Here are three train-ride tales that will prove my point.

The first story, *On account of a Hat*, was written by Sholem Aleichem, who many consider to be the Jewish Mark Twain. Here is a summary of the story: Sholem Shachnah (his fellow villagers called him "Rattlebrain"), an absent-minded and almost-successful real estate broker, was on his way home for Passover. It was dark. He was tired after two sleepless nights. And still, he had to spend a full night waiting at the station for the train.

The only spot available was a narrow space on a bench beside an official who was dressed in a uniform decorated with many buttons. He also wore a military cap with a red band and visor. 'Buttons,' as Sholem nicknamed the man, was lying down on the bench stretched out and snoring loudly. Should Sholem – a Jew in Eastern Europe, in the 19th century – dare sit next to Buttons, a gentile in a position of power, and possibly an antisemite?

Sholem sat down at the corner of the bench, and before long, he fell asleep. When he woke up, still half-asleep and confused, and in a hurry, for he thought he would miss the train, he reached for his hat under the bench.

Instead of his own hat, he picked up Buttons' hat. He put it on and rushed to the ticket window.

The ticket window was crowded, but everyone waiting in line saw the hat and made way for Sholem. The ticket agent at the window asked: "Where to, your Excellency?"

And when Sholem tried to board the crowded third-class car, the conductor with the lantern called, "this way, your Excellency!" and directed him into the first-class carriage. The conductor then saluted and backed away, bowing.

Finally alone, in the first-class carriage, Sholem was wondering: First class? Salute? Your Excellency? Perhaps I am dreaming!

When he glanced at his reflection in a mirror on the train's wall, Sholem became confused (his nickname was "Rattlebrain" for a good reason). In the mirror, he did not see himself. Instead, he saw a man wearing a hat with a red band and visor. In short, Sholem mistook himself for Buttons, the gentile official.

But if he, himself, was Buttons, what ever happened to Sholem? Shaken, Sholem ran out of the carriage toward the bench, on which he thought he was still sleeping, to wake himself up so that he wouldn't miss the train.

At that moment, the train left the station. And Sholem found himself alone on the platform. He had missed the train.

When Sholem eventually arrived at his village – late for Passover, of course – everyone "pointed him out in the streets and held their sides, laughing." Even the children trooped after him, shouting, "Your Excellency! Your excellent Excellency! Your most excellent Excellency!"

145

'*On account of a Hat*' is not just another train-tale of transformation. As all good stories of mistaken identity go, it leads the reader to wonder: What if I were a different person? Would the world see me in a completely different light? Would I be treated any differently?

Here is the second train-ride tale:

On the evening of September 25, 1919, Thomas Woodrow Wilson was aboard the Mayflower, the presidential train, when he developed difficulty breathing, facial twitching, and nausea. The event followed a period in which he had experienced worsening headaches, asthmatic attacks, and congestive heart failure.

It was in the early days after World War I had ended. Wilson took a train journey – a grueling speaking tour that was supposed to start in Seattle, follow the Pacific Coast, and continue to Colorado and Kansas – in order to take his case to the people. His goal was to promote the idea of the Covenant of the League of Nations, which he believed would discourage future military conflicts.

President Wilson was only 63 at the time, but not a healthy man: At age 39 (1896), he felt pain in his right arm and numbness along the fingers of his hand. In 1904, he noticed weakness in his right hand. In 1906, he awoke with loss of vision in his left eye and weakness in his right arm.

And so, in 1919, while on a train journey on the Mayflower, it became evident that more of the same was about to happen. The train trip had to be terminated, and the Mayflower sped back to Washington D.C.

Three days after his arrival in Washington, President Wilson noticed a loss of feeling in his left hand. His left arm and leg were paralyzed, the left side of his face drooped. A neurologist diagnosed him with ischemic stroke, a medical condition in which the blood supply to a part of the brain is interrupted. Without proper blood flow, the affected part of the brain is deprived of oxygen and nutrients, and cannot function properly.

In the hours that followed, Wilson's abdomen became distended, and he could urinate only a few drops at a time.

Dr. Hugh Hampton Young, the preeminent urologist, was summoned. In his autobiography, Dr. Young recalled that "the President had gone thirty hours without voiding urine," and that "His abdomen was hugely distended. He presented a sad picture as he lay there with his mouth drawn on one side, and with paralytic left arm and leg. The condition was evidently desperate."

As a urologist, I often see patients with a history of stroke, or an injury to their spinal cord. These patients often sit in a wheelchair, or use a cane, or a walker, to ambulate. It is intuitively clear to these patients that they can't move their arms or legs because of their brain or spinal cord injury. "But why doesn't my bladder work?" they ask.

"The brain is like a light-switch," I tell them, pointing at the light-switch on the wall. "Then, there is the spinal cord that contains many neurons which run like the electrical cords in the ceiling above us, connecting the light-switch to the light bulb.

"In this analogy," I continue, "the light bulb is your bladder. Any damage to areas of the brain that control the bladder, any injury to the spinal cord that transmits messages to the bladder, could result in bladder dysfunction. If the light-switch doesn't work, or if the electrical wire is damaged, there is no light."

The bladder-switch in President Wilson's brain had shut off. Dr. Young had to come up with a solution, but there were no good solutions at the time. It was a time when presidents were taking the train to convey their message (commercial passenger flights began in 1914; the first electronic TV was invented in 1927). It was a time when bladder catheters were rudimentary. And it was a time when bladder catheterization was dangerous, for it could cause a severe, deadly infection (Dr. Frederic Foley invented the indwelling Foley catheter in 1929; Alexander Fleming discovered Penicillin, the first antibiotic, in 1929).

Dr. Young wrote: "it seemed that a surgical operation would have to be carried out through a median line abdominal incision to open the bladder, and relieve the terrific distention. But could he [President Wilson] stand the shock of it? I hardly thought so."

Based on his experience with patients who sustained spinal cord injuries in France during World War I, Dr. Young decided to wait. President Wilson's bladder became further distended, but the bladder neck eventually gave way and urine began to escape through the urethra. Surgery, and subsequent complications, were avoided.

Over the next several months, President Wilson's general health continued to deteriorate. No explanation was explicitly given to the public, and matters of state were managed by the President's secretary, Mr. Joseph Patrick Tumulty, and Edith, Wilson's second wife.

Wilson served out his term and died of another stroke in 1924.

If a good train-ride story is a tale of transformation, so was President Wilson's, for on that train-ride aboard the Mayflower, Thomas Woodrow Wilson, the President of the United States, confronted his own frailty.

President Wilson's dream of a League of Nations remained unfulfilled at the time of his death. It took 21 more years and another world war for the United Nations to be founded in 1945. And wars still abound.

The third and last train story is autobiographical: When I was about 10, my mother took me on a train ride from Haifa to Tel Aviv – a two-hour long journey. We were on our way to a wedding. My father, who worked in Tel Aviv at the time, was supposed to meet us at the wedding. I wore a new, white shirt, dark dress pants, fancy shoes, and a blue tie – "After all," my mother told me, "it isn't every day that your cousin gets married."

About halfway through the ride, I had an attack of extreme hunger. My mother protested: "Shahar," she said, "we are going to a wedding – there will be a lot of food there." But she ultimately obliged, sending me to the restaurant-car to get "something small to eat."

I bought a large hot dog. It was accompanied by a squeezable plastic bottle with a pointed tip and a label that read "Mustard." I squeezed "Mustard," but nothing came out, so I squeezed harder. I heard a loud pufffff sound, as a small clot of mustard that was stuck at the tip of the bottle suddenly dislodged. Then, I could feel the intense smell of mustard spreading through the air, and when I looked down, I saw mustard everywhere: on my new white shirt and on my dark pants, on my shoes and on my tie, and, it seemed, everywhere else in the restaurant-car. I left the hot dog on the table and returned, hungry and yellow, to the cabin where my mother was waiting.

I could tell that my mother was devastated. She even cried a little. She told me: "I told you..." Then she pulled out her Emergency Plans, found a department store on the way to the wedding, and bought a new set of clothes.

We arrived late to the wedding: desserts had already been served and eaten, and my cousin looked exhausted from the ceremony and the dancing that followed.

My father was worried about our late arrival, but when he heard the mustard story, he started to laugh, and then he laughed a little more and kept laughing until my mother and I started to laugh along with him.

Why is this a train-tale of transformation? Because since that Mustard Day on the train, I always search for humor in life's daily predicaments. When it works, I am relieved; when it doesn't – well, at least I tried.

FAIRY CIRCLES

In the Namibian desert, along a 1500-mile sliver of land in southwestern Africa, one can see almost perfectly round circles of bare sand surrounded by rings of tall grass. The circles vary in size from 7 to 49 feet in diameter. The local nomadic Himba people believe that the circles were created by the spirits, that they are the footprints of the gods. They call this pattern – of bare patches surrounded by rings of tall grass – "Fairy Circles."

Modern scientists do not believe in spirits or in African gods, but like the Himba people, when faced with a pattern, they search for an explanation. "What is the cause of the Fairy Circles?" they ask. Then, they take part in long-winded debates, presenting numerous arguments and counter-arguments, each side entrenched in their own position.

In the case of the Fairy Circles, there are two competing explanations. The first is that plants arrange themselves, or self-organize, in specific patterns. They do so by facilitating the growth of neighboring plants and competing with distant plants. The second explanation is that large societies of sand-termites engineer the Fairy Circles by killing the plants in their centers. Scientists believe that the bare circles of exposed sand allow the termites to preserve moisture and to survive through periods of drought.

In a letter to Nature, one of the world's top academic journals, Corina E. Tarnita and her colleagues presented their solution to the long-lasting debate. Tarnita holds a doctoral degree in mathematics from Harvard University and serves as a faculty member in the Department of Ecology and Evolutionary Biology at Princeton University. In a picture posted on the Princeton website, she is standing authoritatively with her arms crossed in front of her and a wide smile on her face. In my search for the causes of patterns in nature – Fairy Circles and rings of tall grass – I wholeheartedly trust her.

Tarnita did not go on an expedition to the Namibian desert. She did not dig into the Namibian sand, and she did not delve into the social behavior of termites in their natural habitat. Instead, she studied low-altitude aerial images of vegetation patterns in the Namibian desert and images from Google Earth showing the distribution of insect nests.

Tarnita made assumptions like: each colony of termites

starts with two termites, a queen and a king; and each colony grows, reproduces, and seeds the rest of the system with new colonies. Tarnita considered such factors as territory area, the shape of the nest, the rate in which colonies grow, and the competition with other colonies. She put all of this data into several equations that look like this one:

$$pi(t) = \iint mP\ P(x, t')\ dt'dx$$

Then she did the math, and Bam!!! Just like that, she proved that the formation of Fairy Circles cannot be explained by the self-organization of plants alone, nor by the activity of termites alone. Rather, both the self-organizing plants *and* the hard-working termites contribute to the formation of the Fairy Circles.

Will Tarnita's research put an end to the long-lasting debates about the formation of Fairy Circles? I think not, for when it comes to patterns, when one dispute resolves, another arises.

On the day after I read Tarnita's article, on my way to work, I saw patterns everywhere: Driving along US 41, I saw the trees and the forest (trees have patterns, forests too); I saw the waves of Teal Lake breaking onto the shores and the icy sand dunes form into crescent shapes; I turned on the wipers and cleared millions of snowflakes from my windshield – they too have a pattern, a six-fold symmetry. And I thought about patterns of other kinds: zebras that count each other's stripes and leopards that cannot change their spots.

When I arrived at the hospital and donned my white coat, I realized that like all doctors, I too have a duty to notice patterns and to detect disturbances in pattern: a spiking fever; unexplained weight loss; a red, itchy skin rash over the neck; an irregular heart rhythm; and a sudden, intense abdominal pain.

Here is a story about a group of doctors, who by identifying a disturbed pattern, were able to make the correct diagnosis:

Adam was 58 when he came to the ER. He told the doctors that for the past 2 weeks, he had experienced high fevers and drenching night sweats. Adam's eyes were yellow, and his urine was dark.

Before I tell you more about Adam, there is something you need to know about the liver. It weighs about 3.5 lbs. It is a seemingly dull, unsexy organ that sits, motionless and without undue drama, in the upper right side of the abdomen. The liver is, nonetheless, a kingdom of activity: its cells, the hepatocytes, perform more than 500 different functions, including the processing of carbohydrates, proteins, and lipids.

More relevant to Adam's case: Hemoglobin is a red molecule that carries oxygen to the tissues. It gives blood its red color. Each red-blood-cell contains millions of molecules of hemoglobin. When red-blood-cells become old, they travel to the liver, where the hepatocytes break down the hemoglobin. One of the products of this breakdown of hemoglobin by the liver is bilirubin, a very yellow compound. Once formed in the liver, bilirubin flows in a dark-green fluid called bile, via a system of delicate tubes within the liver, and then by larger tubes outside of the liver. Some of the bile is stored in the gallbladder, and some drains into the intestine.

Adam's yellow eyes, his dark urine, and a dramatic increase in the bilirubin level in his blood all indicated that something was rotten in the kingdom of Adam's liver.

But what?

The fevers and the night sweats might have been the result of an infection, perhaps a malignant condition that blocked the tubes draining the liver, or an autoimmune disease where cells of the immune system erroneously attacked the cells within Adam's liver, or along the tubes that drained his bile.

But blood tests showed no evidence of any infection that commonly affects the liver, and the markers of autoimmune disease were inconclusive. An ultrasound of the liver and the biliary system showed no blockage along the biliary system outside the liver. What, then, was the cause of Adam's symptoms? It was time to take a closer look.

The doctors prepped and draped the skin along Adam's neck. They inserted a long sheath that passed thorough the jugular vein, through his heart and all the way into a vein that drained his liver. They then inserted small-caliber biopsy forceps and took a tiny sample of his liver – a liver biopsy.

Under the microscope, Adam's doctors saw the typical structure of a normal liver, with hepatocytes, blood vessels, and tiny bile ducts. They also noticed a pattern not seen in a normal liver (it reminded me of the pattern of the Fairy Circles in the Namibian Desert I told you about earlier): cells called histiocytes arranged themselves in a circle, forming a ring around tiny spaces filled with fat. The ring of cells was further surrounded by another flimsy ring of scar tissue. This pattern – a disturbance in the normal structure of the liver – is the pattern seen in Q fever, a disease caused by bacteria called Coxiella burnetii.

Looking back, the doctors could retrace the events that led to Adam's illness: several weeks prior to becoming sick, Adam made a trip to California. Not very far from the place he stayed at, there was a farm in which cattle, sheep, or perhaps goats infected with C. burnetii lived. The infected animals excreted the spores of C. burnetii in their stool. The spores were then carried by the wind, for a distance as far as 10 miles away. Adam inhaled the spores. He could have remained asymptomatic, suffered from headaches, or developed a pneumonia. Instead, he developed an infection of the liver, also known as hepatitis.

Adam was treated with doxycycline, an antibiotic treatment that is very effective against C. burnetii. His symptoms completely resolved, and he quickly returned to a normal pattern of health.

When faced with patterns in nature, I can see order and beauty. A pattern – and, at times, a disturbance in pattern – is, for my curious mind, a call for new questions, an invitation to discover, a key to the truth.

VINCENT AND I

On occasion, when I feel especially bored, I imagine myself meeting with an important historical figure. The most challenging aspect of this theoretical exercise is, of course, deciding whom I want to meet. I avoid villains, for I fear that the association with them, although totally imaginary, would haunt me. Meeting charismatic leaders, fascinating as they may be, carries the risk of blindly following them. Geniuses in the exact sciences are simply intimidating, whereas extremely successful businessmen might not even find the time to meet with me. As the list of my reservations grows, I realize that the process of choosing the right historical figure to meet with is tiresome. To make matters worse, I deliberate not only about the time and place in which the meeting would occur, but also about which person I want to be in this encounter. Exhausted, I am finally left with a single imaginary encounter in my mind. The year is 1890. The place is Auvers, just north of Paris, France. I would meet with the famous Dutch painter, Vincent Van Gogh. At that meeting, I would assume the identity I feel most comfortable in, that of a doctor – or to be precise, Vincent Van Gogh's doctor, Dr. Paul Gachet.

Vincent was an enigmatic antihero with a tortured soul and a stroke of genius. His early adulthood was a book full of unsuccessful chapters, with attempts to become a bookseller, an art dealer, and a preacher. All of these attempts failed. His love was naive and always unrequited. His behavior was often bizarre: passionate about color, he nibbled at his paints, then ate them; and in 1888, famously, he cut off a part of his ear. Vincent's behavior could have been the result of a mental disorder, perhaps bipolar disorder, but it is strongly believed that he actually suffered from temporal lobe epilepsy. To his contemporaries, though, Vincent was just a deeply-disturbed, bedeviled madman.

In 1890, on the advice of his close brother Theo, Vincent moved to Auvers, where Paul Gachet—a doctor known for attending to artists such as Pissarro, Manet, Renoir and Cezanne—could take care of him.

After their first meeting, Vincent wrote to his brother Theo: "[Dr. Gachet] is sicker than I am ... when one blind man leads another blind man, don't they both fall into the ditch?" But soon thereafter, Gachet earned Vincent's trust, the way doctors often do: "[he] has shown me much sympathy," Vincent wrote in a letter to his brother, and "Father Gachet is very much like you [Theo] and me... he will work with you and me to the best of his power... for the love of art, for art's sake."

In my imaginary encounter with Vincent, I, Paul Gachet, am posing in front of Vincent in my garden in Auvers. He is holding a palette of yellows, reds, and blues, peeking at me from behind the easel, hitting the canvas in short, violent strokes. When the Portrait of Dr. Gachet is completed, I see a work of a genius. In the picture, I am sitting at the table, wearing a blue coat and a yellow hat, leaning my head against my right arm and looking directly at the audience. My expression is that of a compassionate, melancholic listener. In Vincent's words: "sad but gentle, yet clear and intelligent," and "the heartbroken expression of our time." And on the table, in front of me, the solution to human misery: two medical books and the purple medicinal herb, foxglove (Digitalis purpurea), from which digitalis, an important heart medicine, is extracted. So why are my eyes worried? Why is my face furrowed with concern? Is my portrait a mere reflection of Vincent's own tormented soul?

*It is Vincent's tormented soul that I, as his doctor, want to reach. I wonder if knowing more about his disease, temporal lobe epilepsy, would bring some peace to his mind. When I look closely at my own portrait, the Portrait of Dr. Gachet, I realize that explaining what temporal lobe epilepsy is to Vincent, a 19th century artist, may be easier than I thought, for Vincent already **feels** what cells* are: in my portrait, my face is not a whole, but rather a complex composition made of small brush strokes at different hues, sizes, and intensities. I want to tell Vincent that like the strokes in my portrait, our bodies and our brains are composites built from cells.

I want to tell Vincent that his condition may be the result of only a few overly excited cells that reside within the temporal lobe of his brain. They are a group of violent drunks that start a brawling fight in a crowded bar, I would say, cells that are sending the wrong message at the wrong time, generating tiny, yet powerful electrical currents, communicating with neighboring cells, and creating havoc, a chaos of imaginary visions, smells, and sounds. Could Vincent believe that a few cells in his brain were the reason for his devastating experience of alternating excitement and depression, his sudden fury in response to the most trivial of events, his moments of rage and vivid hallucinations? I want to tell Vincent that he is not at fault for his behavior, that he is merely a victim of a few brain cells that have run amok.

Then, in a moment of reflection, I wonder whether Vincent is interested in all that, whether he would find solace in science. Judging from the intensity, the depth, the beauty of his paintings, and from what I have learned about the man, I realize that Vincent **feels** the all-encompassing truth better than any scientist could ever **know** even a part of it. I realize that understanding the science behind his disease would not change how he feels about it and about himself.

So, I leave him be.

One summer day in July of 1890, a fateful shot was fired. It is still in doubt whether Vincent committed suicide, or whether he was shot by another, for there was no eyewitness, and the pistol was never found.

I imagine that the shot was fired under intense blue skies. It abruptly disturbed the silence and disappeared without the slightest of echoes. The crows hovering above dispersed, then regrouped. It happened on a dead-end path traversing a field of bright, yellow wheat.

The shot did not kill Vincent, as he was able to walk back to his house at the Ravoux Inn. Doctor Gachet arrived at the scene as soon as he heard about the incident. He joined another physician, Dr. Mazery, who was already there.

We find Vincent with a small bullet hole just below his ribs. He is holding his wound, his blood – red, dark red – slowly trickling between his fingers onto the wooden floor. He is still lucid, smoking his pipe. He seems surprisingly calm. He is expressing his wish for his belly to be cut open, for the bullet to be removed. I ask myself: can I perform surgery? Can I save Vincent's life? My heart is pounding hard and fast as hell. And I think: it is 1890, it is rural France. And Paris, where surgical theaters are available, is far away. Vincent would never survive the trip, let alone surgery. I carefully dress the wound. Perhaps his internal bleeding will magically stop.

Vincent stayed in his bedroom at the Ravoux Inn. He died on the evening of July 29, 1890. Vincent's last words were: "The sadness will last forever."

IN THE COMPANY OF DEAD WRITERS

There are good writers, and then there are *very* good writers, and then – at a higher level still, in a category of their own – there are writers so revered that the story of their death is told by other writers.

In a story called *Errand*, Raymond Carver, an American writer known for his minimalistic style and moving short stories, described the last days in the life of a Russian writer who happened to be a doctor, Anton Chekhov.

The story Carver told goes something like this: Imagine an evening in 1897. Chekhov was enjoying himself in a restaurant, when suddenly blood began gushing from his mouth.

As a doctor, Chekhov must have known this was

an ominous sign of tuberculosis, a disease caused by mycobacteria (a type of bacteria). Years earlier, mycobacteria invaded Chekhov's body inconspicuously, transmitted from a person already infected with tuberculosis. The mycobacteria might have been released by coughing, sudden sneezing, or perhaps even singing, and then delivered into Chekhov's lungs in a cloud-like droplet of moisture. Once the mycobacteria gained entry, they invaded the cells that were supposed to guard against infectious agents (alveolar macrophages). They lived and multiplied. They did so slowly, but relentlessly.

Chekhov's immune system was trying to combat the invaders, but fell short. He coughed all the time. His temperature spiked. He had chills and night sweats. He had no appetite. He was thin and frail and his eyes were sunken.

Carver tells us that Chekhov "spoke with seeming conviction of the possibility of improvement," but as a doctor, he must have known that his end was near – prior to being diagnosed with tuberculosis (also called consumption), Chekhov wrote: "When a peasant has consumption, he says, 'There is nothing I can do. I'll go off in the spring with the melting of the snow.'"

Carver tells us that Chekhov moved to a spa in the Black Forest with his wife Olga Knipper, and that when his condition deteriorated, his doctor, Dr. Schwöhrer, who quickly realized the gravity of Chekhov's situation, took an action that was "so entirely appropriate it [seemed] inevitable": he ordered a bottle of the hotel's best champagne. Chekhov drank from the champagne. "A minute later, his breathing stopped," and then, "there was only beauty, peace, and the grandeur of death."

Regarding the demise of another writer whom I revere, I will tell you this: Isaac Babel was born a Jew in Odessa, in 1894, and hence, through no fault of his own, he immediately became a member of a persecuted minority. Babel had a tendency to position himself ever closer to death: he became a passionate partisan in the Russian Revolution, worked briefly with the secret police, fought with the Red Army, signed on with a regiment of the brutal Cossacks fighting in Poland, and perhaps most dangerously, had an affair with none other than the wife of the head of the NKVD (Soviet secret police organization). In his final days, Babel was arrested, beaten, tortured, and falsely accused of spying. In 1940, Babel was sentenced to death by firing squad; his body was thrown to a communal grave. He was 45.

Babel's writings should be an inspiration to aspiring writers. In his wonderful short story, Guy de Maupassant, Babel has this to say about the writing of fiction: ''No iron can pierce the heart with such force as a period put just at the right place.''

Why did Babel write a story about Guy de Maupassant? Because he revered Guy de Maupassant as the master of the French short story. And how does Babel describe the demise of Guy de Maupassant? Babel writes: "He [Guy de Maupassant] fought the disease with all the potency and vitality he had. In the beginning, he suffered from headaches and bouts of hypochondria. Then the phantom of blindness loomed before him ... Paranoia, unsociability, and belligerence developed ... he cut his throat at the age of forty, bled profusely, but lived. They locked him in the madhouse. He crawled about on all four and ate his own excrements. The last entry in his sorrowful medical report announces: ... Monsieur de Maupassant is degenerating to an animal state."

Alone, in pain, and totally mad, Guy de Maupassant died at the age of 42.

What was the disease that caused de Maupassant's madness? And was the Austrian psychiatrist's bizarre plan – to cure the disease by infecting patients with another disease – successful?

Winter. 1881. In a room at the back of a Parisian brothel, the writer Guy de Maupassant and a prostitute named Rachel are having a conversation:

"Tell me, Rachel, what is your story?" he asks. He tucks his shirt under his pants, puts on his jacket, adjusts his green tie, and points both edges of his mustache with his fingers.

"I don't have no story," Rachel says, straightening her dress, "and besides, no man comes here to hear no stories, are they? So why should you?"

"Because I am a writer," he says. "I collect stories the way others collect butterflies. The true stories people tell me are better than the stories I could ever imagine. My job is to write down these stories," he says, "that's all."

"Perhaps if you come back," she tells him, "I tell stories only to my regulars." She smiles at him and kisses him on the cheek. "Perhaps next week?"

The following week. Same place. De Maupassant asks for the same girl, for "Rachel, the short girl with eyes as black as ink."

They kiss. She tastes of cigarettes, perfume, and wine. He touches her gently. He puts his ear to her breast and listens as her breathing quickens, as her heart races.

She feels he is not like the men who frequent the establishment. Minutes later, they lie in bed facing each other. He lights a cigarette and pulls at it. "I am a regular now, aren't I?" he asks.

She tells him her story: "It was a decade ago," she says, "at the end of the war with the Prussians. The Prussian army took over Urville. The count of the Chateau d'Urville was forced out, and a bunch of soldiers were living in the chateau. I and a few other working girls were called to entertain the soldiers. These soldiers were brutes, I'm telling you. They were animals, not men. And to top that, they were drunk, the bastards. We, the girls, were drinking too – did we have a choice? But as the night progressed, I am telling you, they drank even more.

"One soldier in particular – the other soldiers nicknamed him a 'Mademoiselle' for he was slim and looked like a girl – was particularly mean.

"He kissed me. That's okay. But then he bit my tongue. So hard that I could taste the blood in my mouth, you hear me. I told him 'for this, you will pay!' He laughed at me, the bastard. They were all laughing – the soldiers, I mean.

"It wasn't until they insulted France and the Frenchmen that I became really angry," Rachel tells de Maupassant. "They said: 'All the women in France belong to us!'"

"'I am not a woman, I am just a prostitute, and that is all the Prussians want,' I shouted back at him. He, the Mademoiselle, mocked my French accent and slapped me hard, on my face."

"And what did you do?" asks de Maupassant.

She smiles at him and kisses him on the cheek. "I will tell you," she says, "perhaps next week?"

As sex happens, people exchange carnal pleasures, emotions, life stories. Sometimes, though, they exchange agents of infection as well.

It was time for de Maupassant to go back to visit Rachel, when he noticed a small skin lesion on his penis. The lesion was red. It wasn't big, perhaps half-an-inch long. It was firm, particularly at the edges. There was no pain involved, and then, about three weeks later, the lesion resolved the way it came about. De Maupassant was relieved.

Three weeks later, de Maupassant noticed a skin rash on his palms. When he was looking at his reflection in the mirror, he saw that the rash had spread all over his body, along his chest and on his back. The lesions were multiple, red and raised, but the rash didn't itch at all.

He didn't go back to the brothel. He did not see Rachel. He just waited. Several weeks later, his rash resolved the way it came about. De Maupassant was relieved.

A good doctor at the time would have easily identified the signs of the disease de Maupassant had. He would call it the "Italian Disease" (the French called it the "Italian Disease"; the Italians called it the "French Disease"; nobody wanted to take ownership), or just 'syphilis'. A good doctor would have suggested applying some mercury to the penile lesion and later to the rash. Mercury wasn't effective – it merely entertained the patient, keeping him busy, while the disease continued to progress.

Several weeks later, when de Maupassant saw Rachel again, she told him the rest of her story: "I got angry at the the Mademoiselle," Rachel said, "and I could not stop myself. I took a knife from the dinning table, and I stabbed the bastard deep in the neck. Blood was gushing from the bastard's neck like water coming from a fountain. Three of the soldiers were rushing to help Mademoiselle. Others were approaching me, trying to hold my arm, but I broke off their grasp, and I stepped back, and I turned away, and I ran, and I jumped through the window into the night.

"They were looking for me for three days and three nights, the Prussian soldiers, but they could never find me. I hid in the church, until the Prussians left town, and tolled the bells of the church every day, so everyone in the village would know how proud I was to be a Frenchwoman, how proud the French people are."

"You said you had no story, and look what a great story you had," Guy de Maupassant told Rachel. "I bet everyone would love to read your story," he said, getting up from his chair.

"Aren't you going to stay?" she asked.

"Perhaps next week," he said. And she knew they would never meet again.

There was no cure for syphilis at the time. The bacteria causing it, Treponema pallidum, was not yet discovered. But the progression of the disease followed a chronicle of a death foretold. In de Maupassant's body, the disease progressed to its final stage, where it attacked his central nervous system. "He fought the disease with all the potency and vitality he had." But in the end, as Babel wrote, "They locked him in the madhouse. He crawled about on all four and ate his own excrements. The last entry in his sorrowful medical report announces: ... Monsieur de Maupassant is degenerating to an animal state."

Then, de Maupassant died in 1893, at the age of 42.

Extreme maladies sometimes call for extreme remedies. And the Austrian psychiatrist's bizarre plan – to cure syphilis by infecting his patients with another disease – was extreme indeed. Did the Austrian psychiatrist's plan work out?

The Extraordinary Professor considered himself an island of sanity surrounded by madness. He was Dr. Julius Wagner-Jauregg, a psychiatrist, a man with an intense look in his eyes and a finely-combed mustache, a man who entertained daring ideas others would consider crazy.

When Julius became the Director of the Clinic for Psychiatry and Nervous Diseases in Vienna, he quickly realized the situation was dire: almost half of his patients suffered from the late stage of syphilis. Some of these patients developed delusions of grandeur. When Julius entered the clinic that morning, for example, he noticed one patient sitting on the floor, holding his head in his hands, his knees folded, whispering: "I am Ferdinand, the Emperor of Austria." Julius knew that the man was a former banker whose name was Fritz.

Some of Julius' patients were euphoric, some were depressed, others were manic. Their neighbors and their relatives brought them to the asylum, sometimes in the middle of the night. And they remained institutionalized. They developed paralysis and dementia. They were all destined to die a miserable death.

Years before, Julius had observed a woman that was miraculously cured of severe psychosis after an attack of erysipelas (a skin infection often accompanied by high fever). Julius designed a grand plan to cure the late stage of syphilis by infecting his patients with a different fever-causing disease: malaria.

In 1917, Julius heard of a soldier that was diagnosed with malaria.

Here is what happened to the soldier before he met Julius: a female Anopheles mosquito bit the soldier in the neck. Some of the mosquito's saliva entered the soldier's bloodstream. Thousands of microscopic parasites called Plasmodium were living in the saliva of the mosquito. The parasites traveled through the soldier's blood and infected his liver, then his red blood cells, where they multiplied and matured. The soldier's red blood cells then burst, releasing a large number of parasites that then entered other red blood cells. This process repeated itself several times. With each cycle, more red blood cells became infected and more parasites were released.

Each time the parasites escaped the red blood cells, the soldier experienced waves of chills, high fever, and profuse sweating. These waves came about in an orderly fashion, every 36 hours. The soldier was exhausted. Without treatment, he would have died. His doctor spoke with Julius and informed him of the soldier's condition.

Here is what happened after the soldier met with Julius: Julius drew a small sample of blood from the soldier. He hoped that the sample would contain enough of the malaria parasite to induce infection in his patients. He injected a small portion of the soldier's blood sample into nine of his patients. He observed them as they developed the signs and symptoms of malaria: chills and high fever. And after several days, he treated them with quinine for their malaria and with Neosalvarsan for their syphilis. Two of the patients made full recoveries and were able to return to their homes and to their jobs. Four others demonstrated considerable, yet temporary improvement. Two were transferred to an asylum, and one died.

These were encouraging results. Julius continued his efforts, and by 1921, he published an article reporting on more than 200 patients he had treated in a similar manner. Fifty of these 200 patients had recovered sufficiently to return to their work.

In 1927, Dr. Julius Wagner-Jauregg was the first psychiatrist awarded the Nobel prize in Physiology or Medicine for his malarial treatment of neurosyphilis. Psychiatrists around the world rushed to replicate his results.

The legacy of Julius is not celebrated. There are three reasons for that: First, because his experiments with fever therapy were conducted on non-consenting patients. Second, because of Julius' personal beliefs: he was an anti-Semite and a supporter of the Nazi movement (although his membership application to the Nazi party was rejected, twice, because his first wife was Jewish). And third, because penicillin was discovered (in 1928, by Alexander Fleming).

Penicillin is still the first line of therapy for all stages of syphilis – a remedy for the primary lesion on the penis, the disseminated skin rash, and the neurological malady that could drive even the best of writers mad.

As I counted the different ways in which the writers I love most have died – Anton Chekhov, Isaac Babel, Guy de Maupassant – I wondered why I bother to tell their stories. I realized that this is part of a larger question: why I write. Perhaps I write to satisfy the need to communicate – a cry into a dark alley in the hope that I hear more than my own echo. Perhaps I write in an attempt to better understand life, death, and other trivial matters. Perhaps the driving force behind my writing is the comforting thought that when I join the company of dead writers, my own children and the children of others will be able to read my deepest thoughts, in my own words.

NOTES ON SOURCES

BEETHOVEN'S EARS

Karmody, Collin S., and Edgar S. Bachor. "The Deafness of Ludwig Van Beethoven: an Immunopathy." *Otology & Neurotology* 26, no. 4 (2005), 809-814. doi:10.1097/01.mao.0000178149.36881.df.

Saccenti, E., A. K. Smilde, and W. H. Saris. "Beethoven's deafness and his three styles." *BMJ* 343, no. dec20 3 (2011), d7589-d7589. doi:10.1136/bmj.d7589.

Argonne National Laboratory. "Argonne Researchers Confirm Lead In Beethoven's Illness." ScienceDaily. www.sciencedaily.com/releases/2005/12/051207211035.htm (accessed January 5, 2018).

LONGEVITY

Sebastiani, P. "Genetic Signatures of Exceptional Longevity in Humans." *Science*, 2010. doi:10.1126/science.1190532.

DRAGONFLY

Arntz, Gerd. „How Long Do Animals Live?" *Compton's Pictured Encyclopedia*. 1939. https://books.google.com/books?isbn=9064507635.

Woolf, Virginia. *The Death of the Moth and Other Essays*. Adelaide: The University of Adelaide Library, 2002.

LIGHT AT THE END OF THE TUNNEL

Borjigin, J., U. Lee, T. Liu, D. Pal, S. Huff, D. Klarr, J. Sloboda, J. Hernandez, M. M. Wang, and G. A. Mashour. "Surge of neurophysiological coherence and connectivity in the dying brain." *Proceedings of the National Academy of Sciences* 110, no. 35 (2013), 14432-14437. doi:10.1073/pnas.1308285110.

IS LIFE TOO LONG?

Emanuel, Ezekiel J. "Why I Hope to Die at 75." *The Atlantic*, October 2014.

Bliss, Michael. *William Osler: A Life in Medicine*. New York: Oxford University Press, 2007.

Heimlich, Henry J. "Pop Goes the Cafe Coronary." *Emergency Medicine*, June 1974.

Shortell, David. "Henry Heimlich, 96, uses his maneuver to save woman." CNN. Last modified May 27, 2016. http://www.cnn.com/2016/05/27/us/heimlich-inventor-uses-maneuver/index.html.

Peled, Smadar. "The Book of Life: holocaust survivors fulfill a dream after 70 years." *Arutz 10 (Channel 10)*, December 31, 2015. http://www.10.tv.

This article and accompanying video are in Hebrew.

Sacks, Oliver. *Gratitude*. New York: Alfred A. Knopf, 2016.

THE TWINS' DILEMMA

Cummings, Brian M., Michael S. Gee, Oscar J. Benavidez, Erik S. Shank, Branko Bojovic, Kevin A. Raskin, and Allan M. Goldstein. "Case 33-2017." *New England Journal of Medicine* 377, no. 17 (2017), 1667-1677. doi:10.1056/nejmcpc1706105.

Thomson, Judith J. "The Trolley Problem." *The Yale Law Journal* 94, no. 6 (1985), 1395. doi:10.2307/796133.

DORA MARR AND CAT

Roberts, Rachel. "Chinese doctors successfully transplant ear they grew on man's arm." *Independent*, April 2, 2017. http://Independent.co.uk. www.sothebys.com/en/sales-series/2012/hong-kong-autumn-sales-2012/-.html

JUST A CUT

Scully, Eileen P., Brandon E. Earp, Amy L. Miller, and Joseph Loscalzo. "Just a Cut." *New England Journal of Medicine* 375, no. 18 (2016), 1780-1786. doi:10.1056/nejmcps1512793.

RATS IN PANTS

Werner Forssmann - Biographical". *Nobelprize.org.* Nobel Media AB 2014. Web. 6 Jan 2018. http://www.nobelprize.org/nobel_prizes/medicine/laureates/1956/forssmann-bio.html

"Charles B. Huggins - Biographical". *Nobelprize.org.* Nobel Media AB 2014. Web. 6 Jan 2018. http://www.nobelprize.org/nobel_prizes/medicine/laureates/1966/huggins-bio.html

"The 2016 Ig Nobel Prize Winners." Last modified September 24, 2016. https://www.improbable.com/ig/winners/?

Shafik, A. "An experimental study on the effect of different types of textiles on conception." *Journal of Obstetrics and Gynaecology* 28, no. 2 (2008), 213-216. doi:10.1080/01443610801912535.

THE MAN WHO SWALLOWED A FISH

New York Times. "National News Briefs; Man Chokes to Death In Effort to Beat a Dare." January 30, 1998. http://www.nytimes.com/1998/.../national-news-briefs-man-chokes-to-death-in-effort-to-beat-...

www.darwinawards.com.

Lendrem, B. A., D. W. Lendrem, A. Gray, and J. D. Isaacs. "The Darwin Awards: sex differences in idiotic behaviour." *BMJ* 349, no. dec10 20 (2014), g7094-g7094. doi:10.1136/bmj.g7094.

ALBERT'S PAIN

Drachman, Douglas E., David M. Dudzinski, Matthew P. Moy, Carlos Fernandez-del Castillo, and Jonathan H. Chen. "Case 27-2017. A 32-Year-Old Man with Acute Chest Pain." *New England Journal of Medicine* 377, no. 9 (August 2017), 874-882.

THE AVIATORS

Barton, Matthias, Johannes Gruntzig, Marc Husmann, and Josef Rosch. "Balloon Angioplasty – The Legacy of Andreas Gruntzig, M.D. (1939– 1985)." *Frontiers in Cardiovascular Medicine* 1 (2014). doi:10.3389/fcvm.2014.00015.

Fowler, Glen. "F. Brantley Scott, 61, Urologist Who Developed Penile Prosthesis." *New York Times*, August 1, 1991, Obituaries.

UNLUCKY STRIKE

Lannoy, N., and C. Hermans. "The 'royal disease'- haemophilia A or B? A haematological mystery is finally solved." *Haemophilia* 16, no. 6 (2010), 843-847. doi:10.1111/j.1365-2516.2010.02327.x.

Dell'Amore, Christine. "Murder of Missing Russian Royals Confirmed." *National Geographic News*, March 2009. https://news.nationalgeographic.com/news/2009/03/090311-romanov-murder.html.

Rogaev, E. I., A. P. Grigorenko, G. Faskhutdinova, E. L. Kittler, and Y. K. Moliaka. "Genotype Analysis Identifies the Cause of the "Royal Disease"." *Science* 326, no. 5954 (2009), 817-817. doi:10.1126/science.1180660.

THREE TRAIN TALES

Aleichem, Sholem. „On Account of a Hat." Translated by Isaac Rosenfeld. In: Howe, Irving, and Eliezer Greenberg. *A Treasury of Yiddish Stories.*" New York, N.Y.: Viking, 1989.

Loughlin, Kevin R. "Hugh Hampton Young at the Bedside of Woodrow Wilson: The President, the Urologist, and the First Lady." *Urology* 100 (2017), 1-5. doi:10.1016/j.urology.2016.10.037.

FAIRY CIRCLES

Tarnita, Corina E., Juan A. Bonachela, Efrat Sheffer, Jennifer A. Guyton, Tyler C. Coverdale, Ryan A. Long, and Robert M. Pringle. "A theoretical foundation for multi-scale regular vegetation patterns." *Nature* 541, no. 7637 (2017), 398-401. doi:10.1038/nature20801.

Geha, Rabih, Marion Peters, Ryan M. Gill, and Gurpreet Dhaliwal. "Histology Rings True." *New England Journal of Medicine* 376, no. 9 (2017), 869-874. doi:10.1056/nejmcps1609391.

VINCENT AND I

Naifeh, Steven, and Gregory White Smith. *Van Gogh: The Life.* 2012.

IN THE COMPANY OF DEAD WRITERS

Raymond Carver, Errand, The New Yorker: 136 , June 1, 1987 P. 30

Babel, Issac, Nathalie Babel, Peter Constantine, and Cynthia Ozick. "Guy de Maupassant." In *The Complete Works of Isaac Babel.* New York: Norton, 2005. (Translated from Russian).

Tsay, Cynthia J. "Julius Wagner-Jauregg and the Legacy of Malarial Therapy for the Treatment of General Paresis of the Insane." *The Yale Journal of Biology and Medicine* 86.2 (2013): 245–254.

ABOUT THE AUTHOR

Shahar Madjar, M.D., M.B.A., is an Israeli-born urologist practicing in the remote, cold Upper Peninsula of Michigan (population 300,000). His medical training took him to different parts of the world: Tel Aviv, Israel; London, England; Miami, Florida; Cleveland, Ohio; Jackson, Mississippi; and Stony Brook, New York. Dr. Madjar is a former fellow at the University of Miami, Clinical Associate at the Cleveland Clinic, and Assistant Professor of Clinical Urology at the State University of New York, Stony Brook. He has published more than 50 articles in the medical literature and has presented his research internationally. For the past several years, Dr. Madjar has been writing a popular medical column for The Mining Journal, and for The Mining Gazette, the two leading daily newspaper of the Upper Peninsula of Michigan. He lives with his wife and three sons in Marquette, Michigan.

Made in the USA
Monee, IL
12 March 2021